**Books are to be returned on or before
the last date below.**

9109

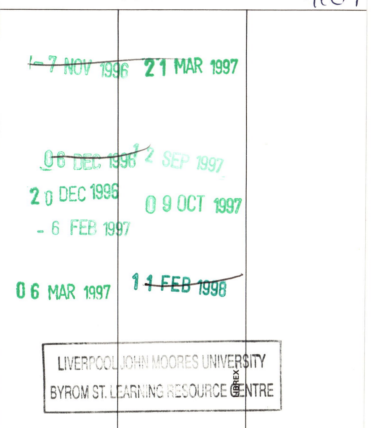

Strain Measurement
in Biomechanics

Strain Measurement in Biomechanics

Edited by

A.W. Miles
Lecturer in Design
School of Mechanical Engineering
University of Bath
UK

and

K.E. Tanner
SERC Advanced Research Fellow
Interdisciplinary Research Centre in
Biomedical Materials
University of London
UK

CHAPMAN & HALL
London · New York · Tokyo · Melbourne · Madras

Published by Chapman & Hall, 2–6 Boundary Row, London SE1 8HN

UK	Chapman & Hall, 2–6 Boundary Row, London SE1 8HN
USA	Chapman & Hall, 29 West 35th Street, New York NY10001
JAPAN	Chapman & Hall Japan, Thomson Publishing Japan, Hirakawacho Nemoto Building, 7F, 1–7–11 Hirakawa-cho, Chiyoda-ku, Tokyo 102
AUSTRALIA	Chapman & Hall Australia, Thomas Nelson Australia, 102 Dodds Street, South Melbourne, Victoria 3205
INDIA	Chapman & Hall India, R. Seshadri, 32 Second Main Road, CIT East, Madras 600 035, India

First edition 1992

© 1992 Chapman & Hall

Typeset in 10½/12 Times by Intype, London
Printed in Great Britain by St Edmundsbury Press, Bury St. Edmunds

ISBN 0 412 43270 6

A catalogue record for this book is available from the British Library

Library of Congress Cataloging-in-Publication data

Strain measurement in biomechanics/edited by A.W. Miles and K.E. Tanner.
    p.   cm.
    1. Strains and stresses—Measurement. 2. Biomedical materials– Testing. 3. Orthopedic implants—Testing.
4. Biomechanics– Technique. I. Miles, A. W. II. Tanner, K.E., 1957– .
  R857.S85S77 1992
617.3'07—dc20   91–25490
                                                  CIP

Contents

List of contributors

Dr M. Dabestani, BSc MSc PhD, Department of Materials and IRC in Biomedical Materials, Queen Mary and Westfield College, University of London, Mile End Road, London, United Kingdom

Dr N. Donaldson, MA PhD CEng MIEE, MRC Neurological Prosthesis Unit, 1 Windsor Walk, London, United Kingdom

Dr J.L. Duncan, PhD, 30 Old Coach Road, East Mains, East Kilbride, Glasgow, United Kingdom

Professor J.B. Finlay, PhD PEng FIMechE, Orthopaedic Research Laboratory, University of Western Ontario, University Hospital, P O Box 5339, London, Canada

Mr M.A.R. Freeman, MA MD FRCS, Bone and Joint Research Unit, The Royal London Hospital Medical School, Whitechapel, London, United Kingdom

Professor A.E. Goodship, BVSc PhD MRCVS, Comparative Biomedical Sciences, School of Veterinary Sciences, University of Bristol, Park Row, Bristol, United Kingdom

Dr A.J.C. Lee, BSc PhD CEng MBES, School of Engineering, University of Exeter, North Park Road, Exeter, United Kingdom

Professor E.G. Little, PhD, Department of Mechanical and Production Engineering, University of Limerick, Plassey Industrial Park, Limerick, Eire

Mr A.W. Miles, BSc(Eng) MSc(Eng) MBES, School of Mechanical Engineering, University of Bath, Claverton Down, Bath, United Kingdom

Dr J.J. O'Connor, BE PhD, Department of Engineering Science, University of Oxford, Parks Road, Oxford, United Kingdom

Dr J.F. Orr, BSc PhD CEng MIMechE, Department of Mechanical and Production Engineering, The Queen's University of Belfast, Stranmills Road, Belfast, Northern Ireland

Dr J.C. Shelton, BA PhD, Department of Mechanical Engineering and IRC in Biomedical Materials, Queen Mary and Westfield College, University of London, Mile End Road, London, United Kingdom

Dr K. E. Tanner, MA DPhil CEng MIMechE MBES, Department of Materials and IRC in Biomedical Materials, Queen Mary and Westfield College, University of London, Mile End Road, London, United Kingdom

Mr S.J. Taylor, BSc MSc AMIEE, Institute of Orthopaedics, Royal National Orthopaedic Hospital, University of London, Brockley Hill, Stanmore, Middlesex, United Kingdom

Professor A.L. Yettram, BA BAI ScD CEng MRAeS MIStructE MBES, Department of Mechanical Engineering, Brunel University, Uxbridge, Middlesex, United Kingdom

Preface

The growth in Orthopaedic Surgery, in particular that associated with the replacement of joints, continues unabated. In the USA and Europe alone, almost 500 000 total hip replacements were performed in 1987. Increasing longevity and high expectations of quality of life are placing increasing demands on the durability of these artificial implants and this is exacerbated by the increasing application to younger and more active categories of patients. However, the introduction of new materials and manufacturing technologies offers scope for continual improvement in the design of implant systems. Regulatory authorities are rightfully placing increasing demands on the rigorous pre-clinical evaluation of these devices. This evaluation is highly demanding since the human body is a complex structure making the measurement of stresses and strains in the body and on devices used in the body very difficult. Bone has both biological and mechanical functions and when designing and using implants it is necessary to be aware of the mechanical influences which the actions of engineers and surgeons have on bone. There has been a considerable amount of numerical work, especially finite-element analysis, done in this area and biomechanics conferences in recent years have been dominated by reports on these studies. Experimental work is, however, somewhat more demanding on resources and, in practice, difficult to apply. There is however a welcome increase in combined numerical and experimental approaches to strain determinations with concomitant benefits to both approaches.

It is against this background that this book was conceived. The original inspiration came from Professor Ted Little who coerced the Editors into organizing a one day Workshop on Strain Measurement in Biomechanics, held under the auspices of the British Society for Strain Measurement at Queen Mary and Westfield College, University of London in March 1990. This workshop was attended by a surprisingly large number of people and thanks to the excellent contributions of the invited speakers was deemed by all who attended as highly successful. In particular Ted Little opened the eyes of all of us engaged in the demanding subject of strain measurement in biomechanics to the appalling lack of technology transfer that occurs between those of us engaged in biomechanics and those who tackle not too dissimilar problems in more traditional engineering fields. How often have problems we confront in biomechanics been solved already and reported in journals such as *Experimental Mechanics*, *Experimental Techniques*, *Journal of Strain Analysis*, and *Strain* (official publication of the British Society for Strain Measurement). Yet, judging by the insignificant references to these journals in the biomechanics literature, rarely do we consult these journals for help in our problems.

This book is not intended to be a comprehensive treatise on Strain Measurement Techniques but, rather an overview of modern measurement methods with particular emphasis on useful reference sources and technical advice on the applicability of different techniques to solving problems. The book is not a proceedings of the workshop but rather a collection of commissioned chapters contributed by distinguished authors who are all authorities in their field. The Editors are grateful for the leverage of their friendship with the authors which allowed them to persuade these busy engineers and scientists to contribute their chapters.

In structuring the book we have attempted to order the chapters with some degree of logic starting off with a scene setting exposé of the general field of strain measurement written by Ted Little and Bryan Finlay in Chapter 1. The inimitable style of John O'Connor in Chapter 2 will hopefully plunge us into the realization of just how complex load simulation is if we are to embark on model testing. The simplifications that engineers like to use of single point loads may well mask important underlying ligament and muscle force components. In Chapter 3, on strain gauge measurement, Ted Little reminds us of the errors and pitfalls that must be avoided and provides a formidable but essential reading list for the serious strain analyst to consult. The importance of seeing how very similar problems have been tackled in traditional engineering applications can only benefit our attempts to improve accuracy in biomechanics measurements. Bone is a highly complex anisotropic material and strain measurements are frequently carried out on cadaveric material. The attachment of strain gauges, and interpretation of data, presents special problems which are addressed by Minoo Dabestani in Chapter 4. There is, of course, almost no more appropriate a test than one done *in vivo*, and in Chapter 4, Allen Goodship brings a more biological viewpoint to the problems and potential of *in vivo* strain measurements in bone. This chapter discusses the influence of functional environment on tissue response in the body and reminds us of the importance of designing and testing implants which maintain physiological levels of stress in the body. Chapter 6 deals with the very exciting prospects of telemetry. Microchip and microfabrication technology has revolutionized such applications and the important data that these techniques yield are highlighted in Clive Lee's contribution to this chapter. Steve Taylor and Nick Donaldson contributed the second half of this chapter and provide a valuable perspective on modern telemetry techniques and developments.

The latter half of the book is principally devoted to whole-field techniques of strain meaasurements. Photoelasticity offers valuable opportunities to model complex geometries to give a first order under-standing of the resulting stresses. In particular, important insights into trabecular bone architecture can be produced, allowing us to better understand how to mimic the load distributions which will preserve normal bone architecture. John Orr in Chapter 7 offers useful insights into two- and three-dimensional photoelastic techniques and examples of applications in biomechanics. Bryan Finlay in Chapter 8 gives an excellent overview of the photoelastic coating technique, which is akin to a whole-field strain gauge approach, highlighting useful tips to short-en our learning curve should we wish to apply the technique. Julia Shelton describes, in Chapter 9, the developments of a non-invasive measurement method, holography, which is a relatively new and prom-ising technique which is rapidly gaining respectability. Lloyd Duncan describes in Chapter 10 how the thermal imaging technique, SPATE, is used as yet another example of non-invasive methods of stress measurement.

The final chapter is a little different in that it does not directly address the problem of strain measurement, but an important numeri-cal method of stain analysis, finite-element analysis. Alan Yettram in Chapter 11 discusses modelling using finite-element methods. When combined with experimental methods, finite-element methods offer great possibilities in optimizing design parameters of implants and helps us to better understand the factors associated with bone remodel-ling responses to prostheses.

We hope through this book that you will be inspired to use some of the techniques which you have not previously considered, either because you were not sure of the pitfalls or advantages or because you were not aware that they were applicable to biological testing. We wish you happy testing and hope that even if your questions are not directly answered in the chapters the extensive references, in excess of 450 are contained in this book, will enable you to find the answers elsewhere in the literature. We also hope that the new researcher may perhaps be brought up to speed more rapidly by having this comprehensive and unique collection of works on strain measurement techniques in biomechanics.

Tony Miles, Bath
Liz Tanner, London

The editors would like to thank John Orr for providing the photographs for the cover of the book.

Foreword

Although the exact physiological mechanisms are unclear it seems certain that bone as a tissue is influenced by its mechanical environment. At one extreme it is known that a reduction in the load applied to bone, for example after space travel or prolonged bedrest, results in bone loss. At the other extreme overload applied either as a single event or cyclically can produce fracture. Load short of this overload may produce new bone formation, as exemplified by subperiosteal new bone production around the tip of a rigid implant within the medullary canal. Between these extremes it is tempting to suppose that the quantity and orientation of bone tissue in a segment of the skeleton depends at least in part upon the local mechanical environment. These relationships are enshrined in 'Wolff's Law'. Although there is doubtless a relationship of this kind within the physiological range of loads, its exact definition has proved difficult since a number of other influences, genetic and hormonal, are at work.

For bone implants (used either to fix fracture fragments or to replace a segment of the skeleton) the impact of the implant upon the mechanical environment of the adjacent bone may well be a critical factor in the long term success of the procedure. Thus it is recognized that if a relatively rigid implant is bonded to a segment of the skeleton, bone loss will occur in that segment. On the other hand, overloading of the tissue at the bone/implant interface in joint replacement prostheses seems likely to be an important cause of loosening and thus clinical failure of the implant.

For these reasons it is imperative that the designers of skeletal implants and the surgeons working with them should have an understanding of the effect of the implant upon the stresses within the adjacent bone. The stresses in bone and interface tissue can be analytically computed using the finite-element technique. Interface pressures can be measured in cadaver experiments with appropriate sensors.

Stresses can be measured indirectly via measurement of strain in bone or the prosthesis. Appropriate pressure sensors (with the possible exception of Fuji film) may themselves interfere with load transmission in cadaveric experiments and therefore in general measurements of strain are preferred. *In vivo* strain in bone or prosthetic material can be measured using suitable telemetering devices and special adhesives to attach strain gauges to living bone. Both these techniques are technically and ethically difficult so that for clinical purposes strains can only be inferred from the X-ray appearances of loaded bones. This is unfortunately an extremely imprecise method so that our present knowledge of *in vivo* strain is dangerously meagre.

Any experimental investigation is as good as the measuring techniques which it employs. Thus experimental investigations addressing the problems of skeletal implants depend crucially upon the techniques by which bone strain can be measured. For that reason the present book is both welcome and timely, bearing in mind particularly the enormous clinical scope for the two fields in which there are grounds for supposing that failure may be mechanical in origin: internal fracture fixation and the prosthetic replacement of joints.

M.A.R. Freeman, London
1992

1

Perspectives of strain measurement techniques

E.G. Little and J.B. Finlay

1.1 INTRODUCTION

Strain measurements in biomechanics are a challenge, even with the established techniques of stain gauges, brittle lacquers, holography, thermography, photoelastic coatings and two-dimensional or three-dimensional photoelastic modelling; however, with care, each of these techniques may yield valuable data. The strengths and limitations of each of these techniques will be reviewed briefly in relation to their potential applications to research in orthopaedics. Applications are quoted from the literature, to help clarify each of the potential concerns or uses. Subsequent chapters provide more detailed information on the individual techniques of measurement.

The most common applications of strain measurement in biomechanics are in product development (Fessler and Fricker, 1989), the evaluation of material properties such as modulus and Poisson's ratio (Wright and Hayes, 1978), the determination of forces and couples *in vivo* (Bergmann *et al.*, 1988) and in the estimation of skeletal behaviour *in vivo* (Lanyon, 1976).

Strain measurements in product development are intended to provide a relative evaluation of orthopaedic implants under static loading in commercial testing machines, in order to:

1. produce data that can be converted to stress and used to establish areas of possible potential failure, which may then be applied to indicate sections for subsequent redesign;
2. reduce material in sections not subject to high stress and thus minimize costs:
3. analyse 'in service' failures;
4. support hypotheses used in finite element modelling.

In mechanical engineering, these measurements are traditionally made by full-field techniques such as transmission photoelasticity (Stanley, 1977), reflection photoelasticity (Daniel and Rowlands, 1973), brittle lacquer (Macduff, 1978), laser holography (Daniel and Rowlands, 1973) or thermographic stress measurement (Thomson, 1878; Harwood and Cummings, 1986). A relative assessment of these procedures, and others are given by Harwood (1984).

Despite the variety of full-field techniques mentioned above, electrical resistance strain gauges (Window and Holister, 1982) are frequently used for discrete measurements. They are not only applied to product evaluation but are also used to determine mechanical properties, forces and couples and to deduce skeletal remodelling. Because of the complexity of biomechanical investigations, it is important that the researcher is conversant with the merits and limitations of the full range of strain measurement procedures. Unless this is the case, he will be unable to select the most appropriate technique, or to identify and quantify the parameters that can bias the results due to the procedure being applied. Many of the problems associated with strain measurement in bioengineering are common to strain measurement in general. Although they are rarely referred to in biomechanics, methods for identifying and minimizing deficiencies in measurements are documented in the literature on the analysis of stress and strain. It is the intention of the authors of this chapter to highlight a few key articles which indicate well established methodologies for minimizing the problems.

1.2 TECHNIQUES

The failure of a material is not necessarily dependent upon simple criteria such as maximum strain or maximum stress; consequently, analysis of the performance of a device may involve the measurement of strains (or other parameters) so that all of the principal strains and stresses may be computed. These values may then be used to investigate various potential failure criteria (Jones, 1975). The following techniques may provide a rapid full-field analysis of some parameter of stress or strain; however, accurate quantification of the data is sometimes tedious and inaccurate. The choice of technique is, therefore, based upon the intended use of the resultant data.

1.2.1 Transmission photoelasticity

Although procedures for applying full-field photoelasticity to product development are well known (Heywood, 1969; Kuske and Robertson, 1977), comparatively few applications of three-dimensional work have been reported in the biomechanics literature (Milch, 1940; Yosioka and Shiba, 1981; Dietrich and Kurowski, 1985). This shortage is probably due to the difficulty in achieving modulus matching in accordance with the laws of dimensional analysis (Hossdorf, 1974) and the thermal expansions occurring at the stress-freezing temperature (Cernosek and Perla, 1970); these are problems which do not occur in finite element studies. Where there has not been a requirement to model the extreme range of moduli in three-dimensional work, photoelasticity has been used successfully for a comparative analysis of press-fit femoral heads (Andrisano *et al.*, 1988), for evaluation of stress concentrations (Fricker, 1990) and for the study of muscular forces which act to reduce the tensile effects of bending in the long bones of the arm and leg (Pauwels, 1950, 1954).

In two-dimensional slices, the isochromatic fringes may not represent the principal shear stress in the original 3-D structure, but may only indicate the maximum in-plane shearing stress (Dally and Riley, 1985a); hence the requirement for deriving all three principal values. Furthermore in two-dimensional analyses stress freezing can be avoided, and materials used for moduli matching in strain gauge model testing may give valuable 'first order' approximations if anisotropy is ignored (Little and O'Keefe, 1989).

It is suggested that two-dimensional finite element analyses should be complemented by photoelastic studies using the closest possible modulus matching. Then, when reasonably similar contours of the in-plane shearing stress have been obtained from both techniques, the moduli in the finite element model may be altered to be more representative of anisotropic materials. This procedure reduces the possibility of gross errors being present in either model and permits the separation of stress to be carried out simply using the finite element package.

1.2.2 Reflection photoelasticity

Coatings may be applied to isotropic or anisotropic materials, either to establish critical sites for the lay-up of strain gauges, or as a procedure for full-field analysis (Blum, 1977). The method for calibration is well established (Measurements Group Inc., 1977).

Problems may arise where coatings are applied to thin sections, such as the ilium of the pelvis, as reinforcement will be induced, which, since the sectional thickness of the ilium varies, will differ, so that results will not necessarily be simply related from point to point. Although it is possible to correct for reinforcement on metals (Zandman *et al.*, 1962), such techniques are unsuitable for materials with directionally varying properties in sections of differing thickness and complex geometry. Lower modulus coatings do not reinforce so severely, but are less strain sensitive (Measurements Group Inc., 1983).

Furthermore, edge effects can arise due to Poisson's ratio mismatch (Dally and Alfirevich, 1969) and variable strain effects can occur through the coating, particularly in regions of high strain gradient (Dally and Riley, 1985b). Analyses of orthotropic materials subjected to transverse shear forces have been shown to induce shear-strain contours which are not coincident with the isochromatics of shearing stress (Kenwood and Hindle, 1970). Moreover, the isochromatics observed with the reflection polariscope are maximum in-plane shear strains which may be of a much smaller magnitude than the maximum shearing strains (Dally and Riley, 1985a). This feature can be checked by observing the contours under oblique incidence (Redner, 1980). The principal in-plane surface strains may be determined from additional data derived from one of the procedures described below.

Where principal strains were required Redner (1963) used an oblique incidence adaptor, but this instrument appears to be unsuitable for use on complex geometries (Chaudhari and Godbole, 1990). Redner (1987) has developed some novel techniques for strain separation but the most appropriate technique is perhaps the stress-gauge, which would be more appropriately called a strain-separator gauge (Measurements Group Inc., 1986a). This gauge can be removed and the model reloaded for further testing (Measurements Group Inc., 1986b). The separator gauge has a gauge factor calibrated for a range of coatings; however, the manufacturers have put a considerable tolerance on the gauge factor since strain gauge reinforcement occurs with gauges mounted onto plastic materials (Little *et al.*, 1990). Chaudhari and Godbole (1990) proposed an alternative procedure for separating strains based on measurements made under oblique incidence but this technique breaks down if there is any inaccuracy in the positioning of the polariscope. When more accurate data are required, it is recommended that the coating be removed by pouring boiling water over it and a strain gauge mounted at each site of interest.

1.2.3 Brittle coatings

A brittle lacquer, when sprayed on a test object and allowed to dry, will display a series of cracks when subjected to subsequent tensile loads. Compression of the sample, during the spraying and drying of the lacquer, permits the sample when unloaded to display cracks resulting from critical levels of compression that existed in the compressed sample (Magnaflux Corporation, 1971). Investigations using Stress Coat (a commercial version of brittle lacquers) have been used to identify critical areas prior to the installation of strain gauges on either isotropic (Macduff, 1978) or anisotropic materials (Cunningham and Yavorsky, 1957; Wootton *et al.*, 1977).

The methodology for spraying on the coating is described by the manufacturer together with techniques for the loading of the product (Magnaflux Corporation, 1971). Calibration bars are sprayed at the same time as the product and are stored adjacent to it. Each load increment on the test sample is accompanied by a test on a new calibration bar to ensure that the temperature and humidity are relatively stable and are not adversely influencing the cracking taking place perpendicular to the maximum principal strain (Cunningham and Yavorsky, 1957; Chaturvedi and Agarwal, 1978), but in composites this strain will not necessarily be coincident with the maximum principal stress (Cunningham and Yavorsky, 1957; Kenwood and Hindle, 1970; Chaturvedi and Agarwal, 1978). Five hundred microstrain is a typical threshold-of-cracking in a uniaxial stress field, but this value is sensitive to the test variables (Hearn, 1971). The coating provides a negligible reinforcement of the model or prototype under test and is easily removed from the surface. A common problem for the inexperienced experimenter is crazing associated with changes in temperature and humidity; the temperature problems may be controlled by local electric fan heaters.

1.2.4 Holography

A conventional three-dimensional hologram is produced by photographically recording the interference pattern between two laser beams. One beam passes by a direct route from the laser to the photographic plate; the second beam is reflected from the object under study to impinge upon the photographic plate. The interference pattern between the two laser beams is thereby recorded on the photographic film. Total absence of mechanical movement or vibration is essential during the exposure.

Holographic interferometry permits the measurement of distortions on an object which has had a hologram recorded at one load and a separate hologram recorded at another load. This procedure is described as double-exposure holographic interferometry. The double-exposure of the two images produces a series of interference fringes superimposed on the surface of the object, the spacing between each fringe represents a change-in-elevation of one-half wavelength of the laser. For a helium–neon laser, the wavelength is 632.8 nm; consequently only small loading increments can be used on most orthopaedic materials. For example, Manley *et al.* (1987) in a study on the femur after applying an initial load of 1350 N, produced interference patterns with an incremental load of only 45 N.

The use of double-exposure holographic interferometry in orthopaedics has been reported in the study of full-field displacements on femurs (Hanser, 1972, 1989; Manley *et al.*, 1987) and fracture-fixation devices (Jacquot *et al.*, 1983; Hanser, 1989; Shelton *et al.*, 1990). An excellent review of its applications in medicine has been given by Ovryn (1989).

A number of other forms of holographic interferometry (HI) have been described as having reduced sensitivity, but are suitable for measuring contours on curved and/or worn surfaces such as total joint implants for the knee and hip. These techniques employ dual-index HI where the refractive index of the viewing medium is changed (Atkinson *et al.*, 1988; Wagner, 1990) and dual-frequency HI where the frequency of the laser source is changed slightly (Hildebrand and Haines, 1967; Atkinson *et al.*, 1988). While holographic techniques provide accurate non-contacting full-field displacement data, the direct comparison with associated strain data is a formidable task (Manley *et al.*, 1987). This latter problem arises, since differentiation of the displacement data is required to yield the information on strain.

1.2.5 Thermographic stress analysis (SPATE)

In 1878, Lord Kelvin (Thomson, 1878) described the thermoelastic effect which produces temperature changes in a body subjected to cyclical stress. If an homogeneous, isotropic material is cyclically loaded in an adiabatic manner, then the resulting cyclical changes in temperature are directly proportional to the sum of the principal stresses at the point of the material under consideration. The technique is currently referred to as Stress Pattern Analysis by Thermal Emission and, consequently, has been dubbed SPATE.

The cyclical loading is necessary to meet the requirements of an adiabatic process and it must be noted that the thermographic data require calibration from some other source. In the absence of known strains or stresses on the surface of the test part, data from a reference strain gauge or photoelastic coating must be obtained from some area of the sample that is under test. Due to potential reinforcement effects of photoelastic coatings and even strain gauges when used on low modulus bone, i.e. below 5 GPa, this calibration procedure is not a straightforward process. Harwood and Cummings (1986) noted that a knowledge of Young's modulus and Poisson's ratio are required to convert the strain data to stress data, i.e. so as to compare the strain-gauge data with the thermographic signal which is proportional to the 'sum of the principal stresses'. Kohles *et al.* (1989) showed a linear relationship between strain gauge data and SPATE signals on a canine femur; the SPATE signals were obtained at 20 Hz between 400 and 800 N but the strain gauge data were obtained with a static load of 400 N, consequently, the question of calibration remains unanswered.

Orthopaedic studies using SPATE have also been reported by groups in Britain (Duncan and Nicol, 1986) and the USA (Oliver and Jaeger, 1987; Samani *et al.*, 1989); however, these people have used a variety of cyclical frequencies, ranging from 2 to 20 Hz, and the reports seem to have failed to answer the question of a repeatable calibration procedure that applies to cortical bone with a modulus as low as 3 GPa, i.e. characteristic of the metaphyseal bone adjacent to implants in the pelvis, knee and hip.

1.2.6 Strain gauges

Of all the techniques described in section 1.1 the electric resistance strain gauge is used most frequently. Many problems associated with the use of strain gauges can be avoided by referring to the recommended procedures for the selection of gauges (including information on backing material, foil, grid geometry, grid size, grid resistance), and for adhesives, solders, lead wires, and protective coatings for short- and long-term applications (Pople, 1979). Practices for surface preparation, installation bonding and installation checking, together with details of common pitfalls are also documented (Pople, 1979; Window and Holister, 1982). More than sixty variables affecting a typical installation are discussed by Pople (1982), and twenty-seven principal sources of instability which can adversely influence strain gauge data are detailed by Pople (1978), together with suggestions for their reduction. Methods exist for noise rejection (Measurements Group Inc., 1980), and reduction of drift (Pople, 1978), with examples of installations where drifting has been reduced to 45 microstrain over a period of 900 days (Freynik and Dittbenner, 1976) and length changes as small as 1 or 2 parts per million detected over a year (Marschall and Held, 1977) in particular situations.

Correction factors for model testing have been defined (Nickola, 1978) which are applicable to general strain measurement, with specific details of corrective measures to compensate for cross sensitivity (Measurements Group Inc., 1982), which is particularly problematic for orthotropic materials (Tuttle and Brinson, 1984), gauge misalignment (Perry, 1969), influence of cables (Pople, 1979), and gauge reinforcement of low modulus materials (Little *et al.*, 1990).

The importance of calibration cannot be over-emphasized, whether by force or shunt methods (Pople, 1982). The authors wish to endorse his suggestion that the strain gauge user should either be able to reproduce the manufacturer's gauge factor by applying the tests defined by Standards, for example, the 'user gauge evaluation' test No. 62 recommended by the '*Organisation Internationale de Metrologie Legale*' or by carrying out an equivalent check. This process is particularly important for the bioengineer working on materials with complex properties, since an inability to carry out competently the gauge factor test on materials with well defined characteristics, has far-reaching implications for measurements taken on non-metallic materials such as acrylics, plastic composites and bone.

In product development (general stress analysis), it is common practice to apply photoelastic coatings or brittle lacquer as a prerequisite to the sensible surface positioning of electrical resistance strain gauges; however, such procedures are not evident in the biomechanics literature. Too often gauges appear to be mounted in areas of little significance, based purely on the researcher's intuition or following in the footsteps of an equally lost soul.

Others widely reported factors in the development of transducers for measuring forces and couples (Bray, 1981) are material selection for the sensing element (Perry, 1983), manufacturing considerations (Dubois, 1974), the selection of strain gauges, lead wires, adhesives and coatings (Pople, 1980), and techniques for compensation, typically of zero shift and span (Dorsey, 1977), single component calibration, for example torsion (Smith, 1977; Bray, 1981) and multi-component calibration (Bray *et al.*, 1990). Techniques for quantifying the uncertainty in the response and the coefficients derived from the calibration are described by Levi (1972) and Bray *et al.* (1990).

Strain gauge work on composites (Perry, 1987) and the quantification of errors associated with these investigations (Tuttle and Brinson, 1984), has implications for measurements on bone with directionally variable properties. Stacked gauges, gauges with stiff backings and stiff protective coating materials appear to have been used successfully by Lanyon (1976) and Carter *et al.* (1980); however, these installations were carried out in thick sections of relatively high modulus material and were validated via appropriate extensiometry. The 'unwary' should not copy these procedures in thin sections of cortical bone, such as appear, for example, in metaphyseal bone, where stacked gauges with high modulus backing may induce reinforcement effects, with each grid affected to a different degree. In such circumstances, corrective procedures are difficult to apply and thus prevent the quantification of principal strains. Non-stacked rosettes and uniaxial gauges with low modulus backing materials are commonly applied in composites research (Perry, 1985) and are more appropriate. Data defining material properties, derived from strain gauges mounted onto thin, low modulus sections or materials with directionally low modulus properties, may also require validation via an alternative method of measurement.

1.3 CONCLUSIONS

Strain measurements in orthopaedics involve some fascinating and challenging problems for the stress analyst. Some of the most common problem areas of strain measurement in biomechanics are also problematic in general strain measurement. In many instances, procedures for identification and minimization of these problems are described in the literature on stress and strain analysis. Where problems do not appear to have been described previously, the researcher is advised to be cautious and be guided by the various potential pitfalls outlined in this text – especially when working with low modulus, anisotropic, or composite materials, all of which are found in biomechanics.

REFERENCES

Andrisano, A.O., Civatti, V., Dragoni, E. and Strozzi, A. (1988) A photoelastic analysis of ceramic heads for total hip replacements. *Second Int. Conf. Engng. Mater.*, Bologna, Italy.

Atkinson, J.T., Burton, D.R., Lalor, M.J. and O'Donovan, P.C. (1988) Opto/computer methods applied to the evaluation of a range of acetabular cups. *Engng. Med.*, **17** (3), 105–10.

Bergmann, G., Graichen, F., Siraky, J., Jendrzynski, H. and Rohlmann, A. (1988) Multichannel strain gauge telemetry for orthopaedic implants. *J. Biomech.*, **21** (2), 169–76.

Blum, A.E. (1977) The use and understanding of photoelastic coatings. *Strain*, **13** (3), 96–101.

Bray, A. (1981) The role of stress analysis in the design of force-standard transducers. *Exptl. Mech.*, **21** (1), 1–20.

Bray, A., Barbato, G. and Levi, R. (1990) *Theory and Practice of Force Measurement*, Academic Press, London.

Carter, D.R., Smith, D. J., Spengler, D.M., Daly, C.H. and Frankel, V.H. (1980) Measurement and analysis of *in vivo* bone strains on the canine radius and ulna. *J. Biomech.*, **13**, 27–38.

Cernosek, J. and Perla, M. (1971) Composite model technique for three dimensional photoelastic stress analysis. *4th Int. Conf. Exptl. Stress Analysis*, Institution of Mechanical Engineers, London, pp. 189–97.

Chaturvedi, S.K. and Agarwal, B.D. (1978) Brittle coating studies on fibrous composites. *Strain*, **14** (4), 131–6.

Chaudhari, U.M. and Godbole, P.B. (1990) Direct oblique-incidence method for reflection photoelasticity. *Exptl. Tech.*, **14** (2), 37–40.

Cunningham, J.H. and Yavorsky, J.M. (1957) The brittle lacquer technique of stress analysis applied to anisotropic materials. *Proc. S.E.S.A.*, **14**, 101–8.

Dally, J.W. and Alfirevich, I. (1969) Application of birefringent coatings to glass-fibre-reinforced plastics. *Exptl. Mech.*, **9**, 97–102.

Dally, J.W. and Riley, W.F. (1985a) *Experimental Stress Analysis*, McGraw-Hill, Singapore, p. 449.

Dally, J.W. and Riley, W.F. (1985b) *Experimental Stress Analysis*, McGraw-Hill, Singapore, pp. 532–60.

Daniel, I.M. and Rowlands, R.E. (1973) Experimental stress analysis of composite materials. *ASME Design Engng. Conf.*, Chicago, Paper 72–DE–6.

Dietrich, M. and Kurowski, P. (1985) The importance of mechanical factors in the aetiology of spondylolysis: A model analysis of loads and stresses in human lumbar spine. *Spine*, **10** (6), 532–42.

Dorsey, J. (1977) Homegrown strain-gauge transducers. *Exptl. Mech.*, **17**, 255–60.

Dubois, M. (1974) Design and manufacture of high precision strain gauge dynamometers and balances at the ONERA Modane Centre. *Strain*, **10** (4), 188–94.

Duncan, J.L. and Nicol, A.C. (1986) Experimental stress analysis of fresh bone using a thermoelastic technique. *Proc. Joint Conf. on Mater. Prop. Stress Analysis Biomech.*, Institute of Physics and Biological Engineering Society, London. pp. 67–73.

Fessler, H. and Fricker, D.C. (1989) A study of stresses in alumina universal heads of femoral prostheses. *Proc. I. Mech. E.*, **203 H1**, 15–34.

Freynik, H.S. and Dittbenner, G.R. (1976) Strain-gauge-stability measurements for years at 75°C in air. *Exptl Mech.*, **16**, 155–60.

Fricker, D.C. (1990) Stress concentration factors for intersecting arrays of notches in beams under pure bending, in *Applied Stress Analysis*, Elsevier, Oxford (in press).

Hanser, U. (1972) Spannungsoptische Untersuchungen bei der Osteosynthese und Endoprothetik. *Z. Orthop.*, **110**, 871–6.

Hanser, U. (1979) Quantitative evaluation of holographic investigation in experimental orthopaedics, in *Holography in Medicine and Biology* (ed. G. von Bally), Springer-Verlag, Heidelberg, Germany, pp. 27–33.

Hanser, U. (1989) Lasertechnische Bestimmung von Verformungen in der Experimentellen Biomechanik, *Labor fur Biomechanik und Biomedizinische Technik*. pp. 629–36.

Harwood, N. (1984) Relative assessment of full field experimental stress analysis techniques. *Strain*, **21** (3) 119–21.

Harwood, N. and Cummings, W.M. (1986) Applications of thermoelastic stress analysis. *Strain*, **22** (1), 7–11.

Hearn, E.J. (1971) *Brittle Lacquers for Strain Measurements*, Merrow Publishing Company Ltd, Watford.

Heywood, R.B. (1969) *Photoelasticity for Designers*, Pergamon Press, Oxford.

Hildebrand, B.P. and Haines, K.A. (1967) Multiple wavelengths and multiple source holography, applied to contour generation. *J. Opt. Soc. Amer.*, **57** (2), 155–62.

Hossdorf, H. (1974) *Model Analysis of Structures*, Van Nostrand Reinhold, Wokingham.

Jacquot, P., Rastogi, P.K. and Pflug, L. (1983) Holographic interferometry applied to external osteosynthesis: Comparative analysis of the performances of external fixation prototypes, in *Proceedings of SPIE – The International Society for Optical Engineering. Vol. 398: Industrial applications of laser technology* (ed. W.F. Fagan), pp. 149–58.

Jones, R.M. (1975) *Mechanics of Composite Materials*, Hemisphere, New York.

Kenwood, K.T. and Hindle, G.R. (1970) Analysis of strain in fibre-reinforced materials. *J. Strain Anal.*, **5** (4), 309–15.

Kohles, S.S., Vanderby, R. Jr, Manley, P.M., Belloli, D.M., Sandor, B.I. and McBeath, A.A. (1989) A comparison of strain gauge analysis to differential infrared thermography in the proximal canine femur. *Trans. Orthop. Res. Soc.*, **14**, 490.

Kuske, A. and Robertson, G. (1977) *Photoelastic Stress Analysis*, John Wiley, Chichester.

Lanyon, L.E. (1976) The measurement of bone strain *in vivo*. *Acta Orthop. Belg.*, **42** (1), 98–108.

Levi, R. (1972) Multicomponent calibration of machine-tool dynamometers. *Trans. ASME, J. Engng. Ind.*, **94** (4), 1067–72.

Little, E.G. and O'Keefe, D. (1989) An experimental technique for the investigation of three dimensional stress in bone cement underlying a tibial plateau. *Proc. I. Mech. E.*, **203 H1**, 35–41.

Little, E.G., Tocher, D. and O'Donnell, P. (1990) Strain gauge reinforcement of plastics. *Strain*, **26** (3), 91–8.

Macduff, I.B. (Ed.) (1978) Brittle lacquer technique, in *Methods and Practice for Stress and Strain Measurement – Part 3 – Optical Methods for Determining Strain and Displacement*, BSSM Monograph, Newcastle upon Tyne.

Magnaflux Corporation (1971) *Principles of Stresscoat Brittle Coating Stress Analysis*.

Manley, M.T., Ovryn, B. and Stern, L.S. (1987) Evaluation of double-exposure holographic interferometry for biomechanical measurements *in vitro*. *J. Orthop. Res.*, **5** (1), 144–9.

Marschall, C.W. and Held, P.R. (1977) Measurement of long-term dimensional stability with electrical resistance strain gauges. *Strain*, **13** (1), 13–16.

Measurements Group Inc. (1977) Calibration of photoelastic coatings, Tech. Note. TN–701.

Measurements Group Inc. (1980) Noise control in strain gauge measurements, Tech. Note TN–501.

Measurements Group Inc. (1982) Errors due to transverse sensitivity in strain gauges, Tech. Note TN–509.

Measurements Group Inc. (1983) Materials for photoelastic coatings, Bulletin S–116–D.

Measurements Group Inc. (1986a) Principal stress separation in photostress measurements, Tech. Note TN–708.

Measurements Group Inc. (1986b) Photostress separator gauge installations with M-Bond 200 adhesive, Instruction bulletin IB–237.

Milch, H. (1940) Photo-elastic studies of bone forms. *J. Bone Jt. Surg.*, **22–A** (3), 621–6.

Nickola, W.E. (1978) Strain gauge measurements on plastic models. *BSSM Ann. Conf: Applications of Materials Testing to Experimental Stress Analysis*, Bradford.

Oliver, D.E. and Jaeger, P. (1987) SPATE applications in North America: Report on US SPATE users group. *SPIE*, **731**, 213–27.

Ovryn, B. (1989) Holographic interferometry. *CRC Crit. Rev. Biomed. Engng.*, **16**, 269–322.

Pauwels, F. (1950) Die Bedeutung der Baussprinzipien des Stütz- und Bewegungs-apparates für die Beanspruchung der Röhrenknochen. Erster Beitrag zur funktionellen Anatomie und kausalen Morphologie des Stützapparates. *Z. Anat.*, **114**, 129–80.

Pauwels, F. (1954) Kritische Überprüfüng der Rouxschen Abhandlung: Beschreibung und Erläuterung einer knöchernen Kniegelenksankylose. Fünfter Beitrag zur funktionellen Anatomie und kausalen Morphologie des Stützapparates. *Z. Anat.*, **117**, 528–52.

Perry, C.C. (1969) Strain gauge misalignment errors. *Instrum. Control Syst.*, **42**, 137–9.

Perry, C.C. (Ed.) (1983) Modern strain gauge transducers – their design and construction Part IV: Transducer spring materials, chapter 2. *Epsilonics*, **3** (2), 6–7, Measurements Groups Inc., Raleigh, North Carolina.

Perry, C.C. (1985) Experimental stress analysis of reinforced plastics. *40th Ann. Conf., Reinforced Plastics – Composites Institute*, Session 5–C., pp. 1–7.

Perry, C.C. (1987) Strain gauge measurements on plastics and composites. *Strain*, **23** (4), 155–6.

Pople, J. (1978) Some factors affecting long-term stability of strain measurements using metal foil gauges. *Strain*, **14** (3), 93–104.

Pople, J. (1979) *BSSM Strain Measurement Reference Book*, British Society for Strain Measurement, Newcastle upon Tyne.

Pople, J. (1980) DIY strain gauge transducers (Part 1). *Strain*, **16** (1), 23–36.

Pople, J. (1982) Errors and uncertainty in strain measurement, in *Strain Gauge Technology* (eds. A.L. Window and G.S. Holister), Applied Science Publishers, Barking, UK, pp. 209–64.

Redner, A.S. (1963) New oblique-incidence method for direct photoelastic measurement of principal strains. *Exptl. Mech.*, **3**, 67–72.

Redner, A.S. (1980) Photoelastic coatings. *Exptl. Mech.*, **20** (11), 403–8.

Redner, A.S. (1987) Separation of principal strains in photoelastic coatings by the slitting method. *Exptl. Tech.*, **11** (5), 29–32.

Samani, D.L., Friis, E.A., Cooke, F.W. and Henning, C.E. (1989) The effect of bone block shape on patellar stresses in ACL reconstruction. *Trans. Orthop. Res. Soc.*, **14**, 215.

Shelton, J.C., Gorman, D. and Bonfield, W. (1990) Holographic assessment of internal fracture fixation devices. *J. Biomech.*, **23** (4), 391 (Abstract).

Smith, J.D. (1977) Practical problems in calibration of torque tubes. *Strain*, **14** (4), 148–51.

Stanley, P. (Ed.) (1977) *Methods and Practice for Stress and Strain Measurement – Part 2 – Photoelasticity*, BSSM Monograph, Newcastle upon Tyne.

Thomson, W. (Lord Kelvin) (1878) On the thermoelastic, thermomagnetic and pyroelectric properties of matter. *Phil. Mag.*, **5**, 4–27.

Tuttle, M.E. and Brinson, H.F. (1984) Resistance foil strain-gauge technology as applied to composite materials. *Exptl. Mech.*, **24**, 54–65.

Wagner, J.W. (1990) Examples of holographic testing versus state-of-the-art in the medical device industry. *Proc. Soc., Photo Opt. Instrum. Engng.*, **604**, 86–94.

Window, A.L. and Holister, G.S. (eds) (1982) *Strain Gauge Technology*, Applied Science Publishers, Barking.

Wootton, A.J., Mackinnon, J.A. and Paton, W. (1977) The role of brittle lacquer techniques in the efficient design of GRP fan blades. *Strain*, **13** (4), 132–6.

Wright, T.M. and Hayes, W. (1978) Strain gauge applications on compact bone. *J. Biomech.*, **12**, 471–5.

Yosioka, Y. and Shiba, R. (1981) A study on the stress analysis of the pelvis by means of the three-dimensional photoelastic experiments. *J. Jap. Orthop. Assoc.*, **55** (2), 209–22.

Zandman, F., Redner, S. and Riegner, E.I. (1962) Reinforcing effect of bi-refringent coatings. *Exptl. Mech.*, **2**, 55–64.

2

Load simulation problems in model testing

J.J. O'Connor

2.1 INTRODUCTION

The bulk of the chapters in this book will concentrate on methods of measurement of strain in bone. Bone forms only part of the musculo-skeletal system; the skeleton is stabilized and enabled to transmit loads by the application of muscle forces. Muscles have two primary mechanical functions; they stabilize the skeleton by preventing movement at the joints and they induce movements at the joints against the resistance of the external loads. Borelli (1679) demonstrated that the lever-arms of the muscle forces about the joints are often smaller than those of the external loads so that the muscle forces can be large, the muscles acting at a mechanical disadvantage. As a consequence, the contact forces applied by one bone to the other across the joints in reaction to the muscle forces are also large.

If one wishes to reproduce *in vitro* a physiological distribution of strain in bone, the experiment should be designed to simulate the physiological application of load balanced by tension forces applied through the muscle tendons. Before discussing the design of experiments, it is useful first to review some elementary concepts in mechanics.

2.2 SOME BASIC CONCEPTS

2.2.1 Loads

External loads are forces applied to the body in one of two possible ways. Loads like gravity are body forces, applied throughout the volume of the body, each part of the body adding its own contribution. When one stands still the weight forces are balanced by the ground reaction, loads applied by the ground through the soles of the feet.

These latter are examples of contact forces, loads applied over part of the surface area of the body by means of contact pressure or friction. Other examples of contact forces are forces applied through the hands when using walking sticks. Weight may be thought of as the primary load, the contact forces as the external reactions to those loads.

When standing still the resultant of the ground reaction forces, the sum of the forces applied through both feet, is exactly equal to the weight of the body. The body is said to be in equilibrium under the action of the weight forces and the ground reactions. When moving, the ground reaction must, in addition to balancing the gravity forces, provide the forces necessary to maintain that movement, so-called inertia forces. When moving slowly the inertia forces are small in comparison to body weight but when sprinting, they can be quite substantial. In the following discussion, it will be assumed, for simplicity, that the inertia effects are small and concentration will be given to the effects of gravitational loads.

2.2.2 Resultant force and moment

The forces and moments transmitted by the joints and along the limbs are internal reactions to the external loads. As an example, consider the lower leg, from the joint cleft at the knee down to the ground. It is in equilibrium under the action of its own weight (small compared to body weight), the ground reaction and the forces applied to the lower leg by the structures of the knee.

The simplest way of describing the forces at the knee or any level along the leg is to calculate the resultant force and moment acting there. Figure 2.1(a) shows the lower leg loaded by the ground reaction W and forces applied at the knee, ignoring the weight of the lower leg. For equilibrium, the sum of the forces acting on the lower leg must be zero so that the structures of the knee have to combine to provide a force which exactly balances the ground reaction. This is the resultant force F at the knee which resists translation of the lower leg. It is equal in magnitude and opposite in direction to the load W. In Figure 2.1(a), the resultant force F at the knee is shown passing through the tibial plateau at the point O. Its line of action does not coincide with that of the ground reaction, although the two forces are parallel. The structures of the knee must therefore also combine to provide a moment, C in Figure 2.1(a), which resists rotary movements of the lower leg about the point O. The magnitude of the moment C must be equal and opposite to the moment of the load about the point O, Figure 2.1(a), the product of the force magnitude W times the perpendicular distance d from O to the line of action of W.

Figure 2.1(b) shows the lower leg sectioned distal to the knee and

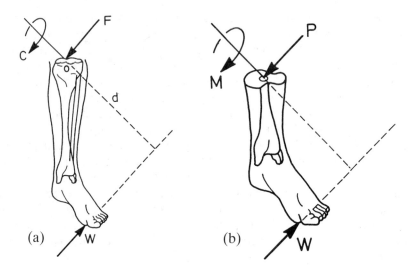

Figure 2.1 (a) The lower leg in equilibrium under the action of a load W applied at the foot. If the weight of the limb is neglected, the resultant force F at the knee must be equal and opposite to W in order to have balanced vertical, mediolateral, and fore-aft forces. If F and W do not have the same line of action, then a moment C equal to Wd (d is the perpendicular distance from W to F) is needed to keep the foot floor force W from rotating the leg (from Biden and O'Connor (1990), Figure 8.1, p. 136, reproduced by permission of Raven Press Ltd). (b) Section through the tibia showing resultant force P and resultant moment M needed for equilibrium under the action of external load W.

loaded as in Figure 2.1(a). The segment of the leg is in equilibrium under the action of the external load applied through the foot and the forces transmitted by the bone and muscle tissues at that section. These forces can also be reduced to a single force acting through some specified point on the section and a moment.

2.2.3 Components of force and moment

The resultant force and moment at the knee can be defined with respect to a coordinate system of three mutually perpendicular axes x, y, z meeting at the origin O, Figure 2.2. The x- and y-axes point in the anterior and medial directions, approximately in the plane of the tibial plateau. The z-axis lies perpendicular to that plane, pointing upwards from the tibia. In general, the resultant force at the knee does not coincide with one of the three coordinate directions but has components in each of those directions. The components in the x- and y-directions, parallel to the tibial plateau, are called shear forces because they resist sliding of the femur on the tibia. The z-component is either a tensile or compressive force, resisting distraction or interpenetration of the bones. The sum of the three components, added according to

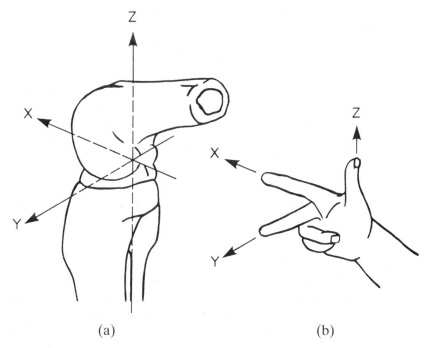

Figure 2.2 (a) Diagram of the knee with axes superimposed; (b) the axes form a 'right-hand' system. The axis system can be thought of as attached or embedded in the tibia. Motion of the femur with respect to the tibia consists of three translations and three rotations. Translation along x is anteroposterior movement, along y is mediolateral inducement, and along z is distraction or interpenetration of the femur; tibia rotation about x is abduction or adduction, about y is flexion-extension, and about z is tibial rotation (from Biden and O'Connor (1990), Figure 8.2, p. 137, reproduced by permission of Raven Press Ltd).

the parallelogram law, is the resultant force, equal in magnitude and opposite in direction to the load applied through the foot.

The external ground reaction does not usually intersect or lie parallel to the x-, y- or z-axes but has a moment about each. The resultant moment at the joint therefore also has three components, one about each axis. The magnitude of each component of the moment is given by the magnitude of the load times the perpendicular distance from the line of action of the load to the corresponding axis. If the load passes posterior to the medio-lateral y-axis, it tends to flex the knee so an extending moment about the y-axis is required for equilibrium. If the load passes lateral to the antero-posterior x-axis, it tends to abduct the knee so that an adducting moment about the x-axis is required. If the load does not pass through the z-axis, it tends to rotate the tibia internally or externally and a corresponding external or internal twisting moment is required at the knee.

In summary, the resultant force and moment at a joint, the joint reaction to external load, can be described and specified by a maximum of six components, three of force and three of moment. The co-ordinate system in Figure 2.2 is chosen so that the components of force and moment are related to the types of movement which they induce or resist. Similarly, the resultant force and moment at any cross-section of the leg, Figure 2.1(b), can be expressed as six components, three of force and three of moment. The axial component of the moment tends to twist the leg, the transverse components to bend it. They are called twisting moments (or torques) and bending moments respect-ively. In any experiment, it is clear that the resultant force and moment at any section of the limb should be known if measurements of strain at that section are to be interpreted correctly. Alternatively, at least six independent measurements of strain at a section are needed if the resultant force or moment at that section are to be deduced.

2.2.4 Degrees of freedom

If all the soft tissues which hold the bones together at the knee were cut, the tibia would be entirely free to move relative to the femur and the two bones would have six degrees of freedom relative to each other. With the femur fixed, the tibia could then slide or translate in each of the three perpendicular directions of Figure 2.2 and it could spin or rotate about the axes in each of those three directions.

Flexion/extension of the knee is a rotation of the tibia relative to the femur about the medio-lateral y-axis. Ab/adduction of the knee is a rotation of the tibia about the antero-posterior x-axis. Tibial rotation is rotation about the z-axis. Antero-posterior subluxation is a trans-lation along the x-axis, medio-lateral subluxation is a translation along the y-axis and distraction of the bones is a translation along the z-axis.

It is no coincidence that the number of possible degrees of freedom of the tibia, six, is exactly equal to the maximum number of com-ponents of force and moment needed to describe the joint reaction. For equilibrium of any body, the sum in each of three directions of all the forces applied to that body must be zero. So also must the moment of those forces about the axes through any point in each of the three directions. There are therefore six mechanical conditions to be satisfied for equilibrium. Six independent forces applied by the muscles, liga-ments and articular surfaces at the knee are therefore sufficient to ensure the equilibrium of the lower leg in the presence of any arbitrary load and to suppress all six degrees of freedom.

2.2.5 Load transmission across joints

The description given above of the resultant force or moment at a joint or at any section along a limb requires no anatomical knowledge and does not specify the structures used to transmit the resultant force and moment. There are some differences between the mode of load transmission at joints and along limbs.

At a joint, the articular surfaces have very low coefficients of friction thus the surfaces can transmit only compressive stress perpendicular to each other to prevent interpenetration. The soft tissues joining the bones together apply tension forces along the lines of their fibres. These forces resist elongation of the fibres and distraction of the joint. It follows that all six components of force and moment at a joint are transmitted by some combination of compressive stress on the articular surfaces and tensile stress in the soft tissues.

At a fully congruous joint like the hip, with two concentric spherical articular surfaces, the bones are free to move relative to each other about the centre of the sphere, a point which remains fixed relative to both. If the line of action of the external load passes through the centre of the sphere, it does not tend to rotate the bones relative to each other and can be balanced by compressive stress on the articular surfaces, without muscle action. If the line of action of the load does not pass through the centre of the sphere, muscle action is required, Figure 2.3. The geometric centre of the joint is therefore also the mechanical centre, the fulcrum about which the external loads and the internal muscle forces exert their leverage. As Borelli pointed out (Borelli, 1679), the muscle's forces are larger than the loads whenever the load lever-arms are longer than the muscle lever-arms. The contact forces in Figure 2.3 are then also larger than the loads. Paul (1967) reported contact forces at the hip more than three times body weight during level walking.

It is more difficult to find the centre of an incongruous joint like the knee. Following Strasser (1917), a simplified model of the knee in the sagittal plane has been presented (O'Connor *et al.*, 1989, 1990c) showing that the instantaneous centre of the joint in that plane lies at the point of intersection of lines representing the cruciate ligaments. The flexion axis of the joint passes through the instantaneous centre. Because the geometry of the ligaments changes as the joint flexes or extends, the instantaneous centre moves relative to both bones and the femur rolls as well as slides on the tibia. The line of action of the tibio-femoral contact force therefore moves backwards and forwards on the tibial plateau while the directions of the ligament forces change. In any position, loads applied through the instantaneous centre can be balanced by some combination of ligament and tibio-femoral contact

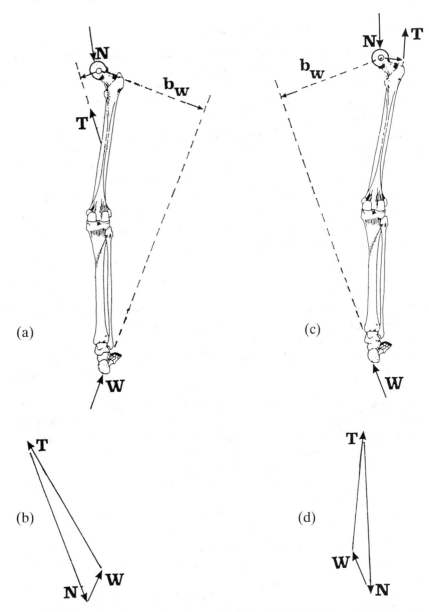

Figure 2.3 (a) The leg seen from the front with a load W applied through the foot and passing lateral to the femoral head. Abduction is prevented by adductor muscle force T. The lever arm available to the load is the distance b_w. Similarly, the lever-arm available to the muscle is the perpendicular distance from the centre of the hip to the line of action of the muscle force. The relationships between load, muscle force, and the intra-articular contact force N are indicated by the triangle of forces; (b), (c), (d) abductor response to an adducting load passing medial to the femoral head. In both examples, the muscle force is larger than the load because the muscle lever-arm is shorter than that of the load (from O'Connor *et al.* (1990c), Figure 10.2, p. 165, reproduced by permission of Raven Press Ltd).

forces, without muscle action (O'Connor *et al.*, 1990b). Muscle forces are required when the line of action of the load does not pass through the instantaneous centre and their lever-arm lengths are measured from the instantaneous centre (O'Connor *et al.*, 1990b).

In reality, movement of the bones at the knee is more complex and three dimensional. It is best described in terms of the helical screw axis of the joint (Kinzel *et al.*, 1972), which takes account of rotations about the tibial axis and possible abduction and adduction as well as the rolling movements of flexion and extension. Loads which do not pass through the helical screw axis tend to rotate the bones on each other and require muscle forces for balance. The lever-arms of the loads and muscles are properly measured from the helical screw axis. Location of the helical screw axis requires measurements of movement relative to all six possible degrees of freedom (Kinzel *et al.*, 1972).

In summary, the large contact forces transmitted across joints are a consequence of the short lever-arms of the muscles and of the need for muscle action whenever the applied loads do not pass through the rotation axes of the joints.

2.2.6 Load transmission along limbs

Figure 2.4 shows a model of the leg in the sagittal plane (Collins, 1990) with hip knee and ankle joints joining the pelvis to the femur, the femur to the tibia, the tibia to the foot. In the model, so-called monarticular muscles span just one joint, tibialis anterior and soleus across the ankle, the gluteus and iliopsoas across the hip. Biarticular muscles span two joints, quadriceps and hamstrings across the hip and knee, gastrocnemius across knee and ankle. The lines of action of all but gluteus and iliopsoas lie more or less parallel to the axes of the bones.

If the line of action of the external load in Figure 2.1(b) were to pass precisely through the centres of the ankle and knee, and if the line joining the centres of the joints were to pass through the centroid of the tibial cross-section at every level, then the tibia would be put into a state of pure compression. The resultant force at any level would be axial in direction, passing through the centroid of the cross-section of the bone and with the same value at any level.

These ideal loading conditions are rarely, if ever, achieved. The conditions of Figure 2.1(b) are more typical where the cross-section of the limb has to transmit shear forces, bending moments and twisting moments as well as an axial compressive force. The tubular form of the long bones between their epiphyses is ideal for transmitting bending or twisting moments. By having the bulk of the bone transmitting the moments as far as possible from the axis of bending or twisting, the

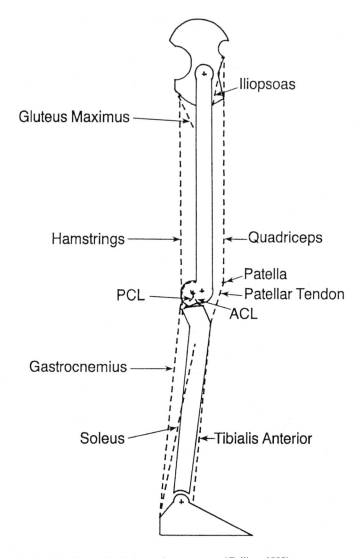

Figure 2.4 Model of lower limb drawn by computer (Collins, 1990).

level of stress in the bone is kept as small as possible. A bar with a specified strength in bending or torsion is made as light as possible if it is hollow. However, the transmission of a bending moment sets up a non-uniform distribution of axial stress and strain in the bone, compressive on one side and tensile on the other. Twisting moments are transmitted by shear stresses on cross-sectons perpendicular to the axis of the bone but these are equivalent to compressive and tensile stresses acting on planes at 45° to the axis (Crandall *et al.*, 1978), such tensile stresses being responsible for compound spiral fractures of the tibia when transmitting excessive torque.

Although the tubular bones are capable of transmitting bending and twisting moments, they can be assisted in doing so by the muscles. As an example, consider Figure 2.5(a) which shows the lower leg in contact with the ground during mid-stance in normal walking when the foot, in addition to supporting the weight of the body, is pushing the ground backwards. The ground, in reaction, pushes the foot forward so that the resultant ground reaction W passes in front of both ankle and knee, tending to dorsiflex the ankle and extend the knee. EMG studies show that both sets of calf muscles, soleus and gastrocnemius, are usually active in mid-stance (Inman *et al.*, 1981). As can be seen from Figure 2.4, both these muscles span the ankle and resist dorsiflexion there; of the two groups, only gastrocnemius spans the knee as well and resists extension there. The lever-arm of gastrocnemius relative to the long-axis of the tibia is relatively constant whereas that of soleus diminishes to zero proximally. Not only do the two muscle groups stabilize the ankle and the knee, they also share in the transmission of bending moment along the leg between the joints.

A sketch of a possible distribution of bending moment along the leg is given in Figure 2.5(b). At the ankle, the dorsiflexing moment of the load is $M_a = l_a W$, where l_a is the lever arm available to the load at the ankle, it is balanced by the moments of the two muscle forces about the flexion axis of the ankle. At the knee, the extending moment of the load is $M_k = l_k W$. It is balanced by the moment of the gastrocnemius about the flexion axis of the knee. Between the two joints, the bending moment in the leg varies linearly between the two values M_a and M_k, at any level along the leg, the moment of the load is balanced by a combination of the moments of the two muscle forces about the centroid of the tibia together with the moment M_b transmitted by the tubular bone itself. The muscle forces and the resultant force F transmitted by the bone form a pure couple. The diagram, Figure 2.5(b), suggests that the moment transmitted by the bone, M_b, is only a small proportion of the total, the large bulk of the moment being transmitted by the muscle/bone couples. Pauwels (1980) gave several examples of the way muscle and tension-band forces can minimize the bending moments transmitted by the bones.

There is a price to be paid for protection of the tubular bone from bending moment. The resultant force at any level of the bone, $\bar{F}$ in Figure 2.5(a) has to balance the upward pull of the muscles forces S and G as well as the upward thrust of the external load W and can be several times larger than the external load. The value of the resultant force in the bone changes discontinuously through the insertion area

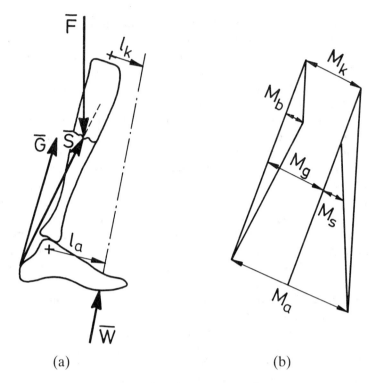

(a)   (b)

Figure 2.5 (a) The lower leg loaded by ground reaction $\bar{W}$ which is balanced by forces $\bar{G}$ and $\bar{S}$ in gastrocnemius and soleus; (b) the distribution of bending moment in the leg, varying from M_a at the ankle to M_k at the knee. This is transmitted in part by the moment M_g of the gastrocnemius force, in part by the moment M_s of soleus and in part by the moment M_b of the bone itself.

of a muscle tendon so that strains measured just below an insertion area may be very different to those measured just above.

If, in a laboratory experiment, the external load acting on the limb is accurately simulated but simulation of the muscle force is not attempted, the entire bending moment due to the load is carried by the bone, the distribution of strain in the bone is entirely non-physiological and the experiment may be of limited relevance.

2.3 APPARATUS DESIGN

2.3.1 Objects of *in vitro* experiments

Apart from studies of the mechanical properties of bone and soft tissue, *in vitro* experiments in orthopaedic mechanics are carried out with a number of objects. These include: to determine the range of movements of the bones at a joint in the presence of various external loads, to determine the roles of the muscles, the ligaments and the articular surfaces in controlling and limiting movements of the bones relative to each other, in transmitting load across the joint and in stabilizing the limb in the presence of external load, to determine the distribution of strain and stress in various elements of the musculo-skeletal system. If these objects are to be met fully, it is clearly necessary that the loads should be applied and transmitted along the limbs and across the joints of a specimen in a reasonable simulation of physiological conditions. The applied loads should be measured in such a way that the resultant force and moment transmitted at any joint or at any section along the limb can be determined. Only then are the mechanical circumstances of the experiment fully defined.

As an example, a description is given in the next paragraphs of an apparatus built for studying the stability of the human knee joint.

2.3.2 Six degrees of freedom apparatus

Most of the six possible degrees of freedom of two bones which meet at a joint are suppressed by the passive structures of the joint, the articular surfaces, ligaments and capsule, leaving only a limited range of flexion, rotation, abduction or adduction. Studies of the passive stability of the joint seek to determine how the passive structures limit the relative movement of the bones on each other. If the passive constraints are to be allowed to act physiologically *in vitro*, it follows that any apparatus used to hold the bones must not itself constrain their relative movement but should allow them six degrees of freedom relative to each other. In the unloaded state, it should then be possible to place the bones in any position within the natural range of movement and they should remain there. When load is applied, any tendency of the bones to move should be restrained by tension forces applied by means of wires sewn to the muscle tendons. The loads applied should be measured to ensure that the resultant force and moment at any section of the specimen can be deduced. Six independent components of movement, rotations or translations, should be measured in order to determine the relative movement of the two bones.

2.3.3 A flexed-knee stance rig

Bourne *et al.* (1978), Biden (1981), Biden *et al.* (1984), FitzPatrick (1989) used a six degree of freedom rig which simulates flexed-knee stance, Figure 2.6. A full description of the rig is given by Biden and O'Connor (1990). The knee specimen is loaded in flexion with stability maintained by pulling on the quadriceps tendon through a load cell. Standing with the knees bent, riding a bicycle, climbing stairs, the

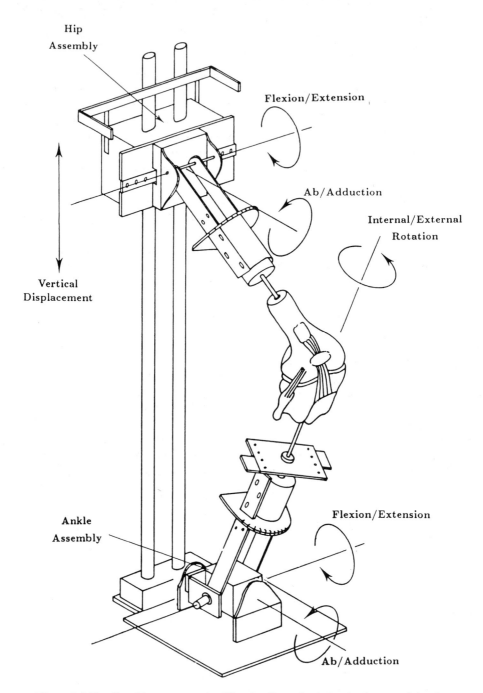

Figure 2.6 The flexed-knee stance rig. The rig allows the knee six degrees of freedom through a combination of three rotations at the ankle assembly, two rotations at the hip assembly and vertical displacement of the hip assembly. When vertical load is applied by hanging weights on the hip assembly, equilibrium is maintained by tension force in a wire (not shown) connecting the quadriceps tendon to the hip assembly (from Biden and O'Connor (1990), Figure 8.13 (B), p. 146, reproduced by permission from Raven Press Ltd).

early stance portion of gait and so forth are examples of conditions that can be simulated in the test rig.

The rig is similar to that used by Perry *et al.* (1975) but their arrangement allowed only five degrees of freedom. A ball and socket joint at the hip gave three rotational degrees of freedom. A single axis rotation was allowed at the ankle and the hip could be translated vertically relative to the ankle to place the knee specimen in various positions of flexion. Under vertical load, equilibrium was maintained by tension applied to the quadriceps tendon.

2.3.4 Ankle and hip assemblies

The specimen is prepared with about 20 cm of bone above and below the knee joint cleft and threaded rods are fixed in the intramedullary cavities of both bones. The threaded rods are used to attach the specimen to the tibial and femoral limbs of the apparatus. The 'ankle' assembly comprises three sets of rotary bearings which allow flexion/extension, abduction/adduction and long axis rotation of the tibial limb. The axes of the three bearings intersect at a fixed point, the centre of the ankle. The 'hip' assembly comprises two sets of rotary bearings, allowing abduction/adduction and flexion/extension to the femoral limb. The axes of these bearings intersect at a point vertically above the ankle, simulating the centre of the hip. Linear bearings running along two vertical rods guide vertical movement of the hip relative to the ankle.

2.3.5 Application of load

When the moving parts of the apparatus are counterbalanced with the specimen in position, the 'leg' can then be placed in any position of flexion and remains there. When vertical load is applied by hanging weights onto the hip assembly, collapse of the system is prevented by means of the tension force in a wire attached to the quadriceps tendon. The specimen is flexed by lengthening the wire. This simulation of muscle force is necessary to stabilize the leg in the presence of vertical load. A strain-gauged proving ring in series with the wire measures the tendon force.

2.3.6 Adjustment in the coronal plane

The bearings allowing flexion/extension at the hip are attached to a sliding bar which can be moved medio-laterally on the hip assembly, thus allowing the plane in which the knee flexes and extends to be rotated about the ankle. When the slider is fixed so that the tibia lies in a vertical plane, this arrangement simulates the natural valgus angle of the femur and the plane of the vertical load then coincides with the plane through the so-called mechanical axis of the limb, the plane through the centres of the ankle, knee and hip. In other positions, Figure 2.7(a) and (b), it allows the plane of the limb to be set at any desired angle relative to the vertical load, for instance to simulate single leg stance, Figure 2.7(b), when the line of action of the vertical load passes medial to the knee (Maquet, 1976 Figure 17).

In the configuration of Figure 2.7(b), the applied load has an adducting as well as a flexing component relative to the specimen. Purely adducting or abducting loads have been applied (FitzPatrick, 1989) by pulling the tibial limb medially or laterally through a system of pulleys, using dead-weight. Similarly, a pure torque was applied to the tibia by means of equal and opposite forces applied to a pulley attached to the tibial limb.

The vertical component of any applied load is transmitted to the base plate entirely at the ankle. The horizontal component in the sagittal plane is transmitted by means of two horizontal forces at the hip and ankle bearings. Similarly, two horizontal components at the hip and ankle bearings in the coronal plane transmit any component of load in that plane. The values of the five components of force can be deduced from the loads by resolving forces vertically and in both horizontal directions and by taking moments about axes in the sagittal and coronal planes. Because of the axial bearing in the tibial limb, all the torque applied about the tibial axis is transmitted across the knee specimen. Thus, the resultant force and moment transmitted across the knee specimen can be calculated by statics from the applied loads. The system may be said to be 'Statically Determinate' and the mechanical state of the specimen is completely defined.

As was mentioned above, knowledge of the resultant force and moment at the joint has to be supplemented by knowledge of the directions of the lines of action of the muscle, ligament and contact forces before the forces transmitted by those structures can be deduced. Figure 2.8 shows the value of the measured quadriceps per unit applied vertical load plotted against flexion angle for eleven specimens (O'Connor *et al.*, 1990c). The solid line in the graph was derived from the model of the knee joint in the sagittal plane (O'Connor *et al.*, 1990b), providing perhaps an upper bound to the measurements. In the absence of a theory, knowledge of the value of the quadriceps force in any position and separate measurement of its direction would allow calculation of the components of force transmitted normal and tangential to the tibial plateau.

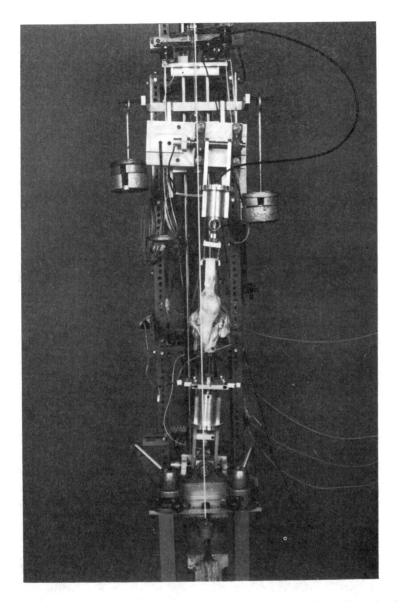

Figure 2.7 (a) Hip slide positioned so that the vertical plane through the hip and ankle passes through the lateral compartment of the knee.

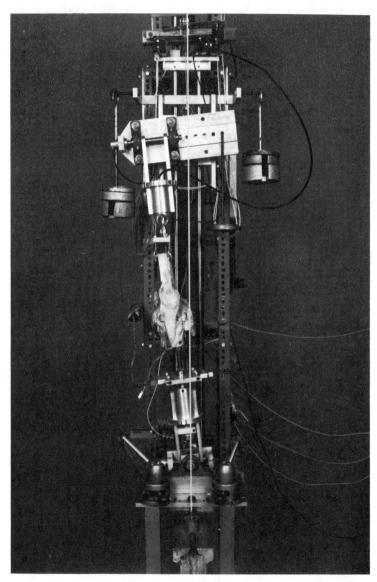

Figure 2.7 (cont'd) (b) Hip slider positioned so that the vertical plane through the centres of the hip and ankle passes medial to the knee (from Biden and O'Connor (1990), Figures 8.14(A) and 8.14(B), p. 147, reproduced by permission from Raven Press Ltd).

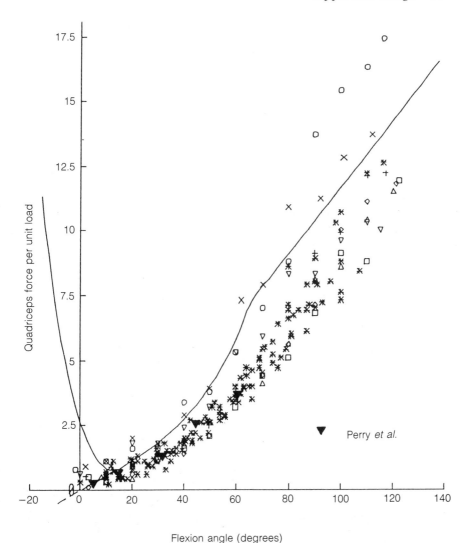

Figure 2.8 Quadriceps force per unit applied load, plotted against flexion angle for 11 specimens in the flexed knee stance rig. Solid and dashed lines were obtained from computer models with and without the contribution of the posterior capsule. Data marked ▼ obtained from Perry *et al.* (1975) (from O'Connor *et al.* (1990a), Figure 12.5, p. 243, reproduced by permission of Raven Press Ltd).

2.3.7 Measurement of movement

Five rotary variable differential transformers (RVDT's) (Schaevitz) are used to measure rotations at the five sets of rotary bearings. A linear variable differential transformer (LVDT) (Schaevitz) is used to measure the vertical position of the hip assembly. These transducers give an output voltage proportional to position. The signals are supplied to a microcomputer (Research Machines 380Z) through an analogue/digital converter and recorded. Records of experiments can then be stored on disc.

2.3.8 Degrees of freedom

Figure 2.9 shows how the degrees of freedom allowed by the apparatus could be combined to give each of the six possible anatomical movements at the specimen, demonstrating that the apparatus does not restrict any physiologically possible movement of the bones. Distraction of the joint and long axis rotation each require movement at only one of the bearings, Figure 2.9(f) and (c), but each of the other anatomical movements requires movement at three of the bearings; for instance, flexion of the knee requires flexion and vertical translation at the hip and flexion at the ankle, Figure 2.9(a), anterior translation of the tibia relative to the femur requires flexion and vertical movement at the hip, extension at the ankle, Figure 2.9(d). Using Cardan coordinates, a program was devised (FitzPatrick, 1989) to express the measurements in terms of the anatomical movements as described in Figure 2.2. Figure 2.10 shows tibial torque plotted against tibial rotation for seven specimens (Biden, 1981) at different values of the applied vertical load and at two different flexion angles, demonstrating how the torsional stiffness of the knee is increased by the presence of muscle forces.

2.4 DISCUSSION

Because the apparatus described in the preceding paragraphs is statically determinate, it reproduces physiological conditions to the extent that the applied loads are themselves typical of physiological conditions. The distribution of forces and moments throughout the specimen may then also be typical of physiological conditions. The disadvantage of having to apply forces through the muscle tendons is that they are very slippery and the magnitudes of the loads which can be applied to the apparatus are limited by the difficulty of obtaining secure attachment to the tendons. Thus, while the force distributions may be physiological, the force magnitudes may be somewhat less than the maximum values encountered in normal activities.

2.4.1 Constrained apparatus

To achieve force magnitudes typical of physiological activities, it is often convenient to use apparatus which applies non-physiological con-

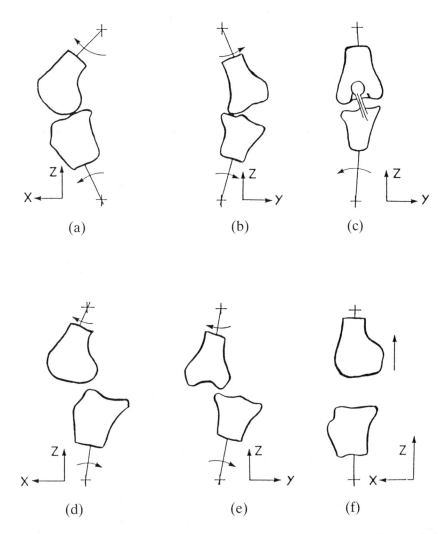

Figure 2.9 Combinations of movements in the rig necessary to give each of the six anatomical degrees of freedom of the knee. In (a), flexion at both hip and ankle with vertical descent of the hip, allows knee flexion. In (b), ab/adduction at hip and ankle, with vertical descent of the hip, allows knee ab/adduction. In (c), a single movement, ankle rotation, allows long axis rotation of the tibia relative to the femur. In (d), antero-posterior translation of the femur on the tibia requires flexion at the hip and extension at the ankle (or *vice versa*) with vertical ascent of the hip. In (e), medio-lateral subluxation of the knee requires abduction at the hip and adduction at the ankle (or *vice versa*) with ascent of the hip. In (f), distraction of the knee requires ascent of the hip (from Biden and O'Connor (1990), Figure 8.15, p. 148, reproduced by permission from Raven Press Ltd).

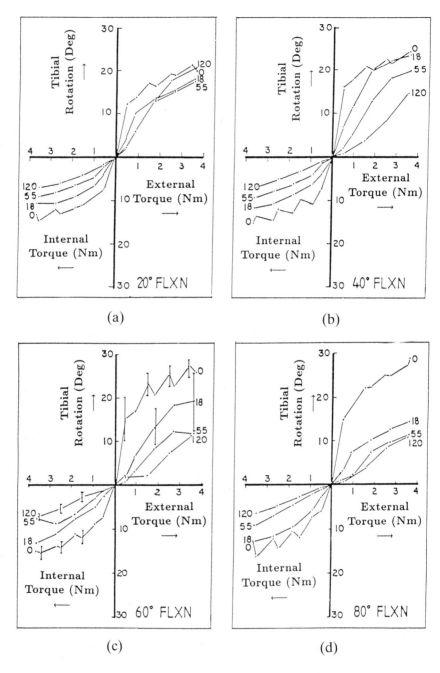

Figure 2.10 Tibial rotation plotted against torque at 20°(a), 40°(b), 60°(c) and 80°(d) of flexion for seven specimens. Results are presented for vertical loads of 0, 40, 80 and 120 N with associated quadriceps forces as in Figure 2.8. Part c contains bars to indicate one standard deviation from the mean of seven measurements (from O'Connor *et al.* (1990a), Figure 12.16, p. 260, reproduced by permission of Raven Press Ltd).

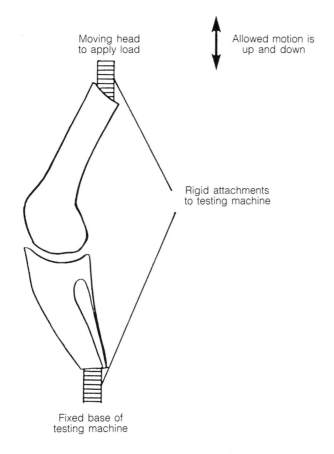

Moving head
to apply load

Allowed motion is
up and down

Rigid attachments
to testing machine

Fixed base of
testing machine

Figure 2.11 The one-degree-of-freedom rig. Bone can only distract or interpenetrate, and motions involving flexion and rotations are suppressed. Also, the knee is held in flexion without muscle activity, which is not the usual case in a live joint (from Biden and O'Connor (1990), Figure 8.5, p. 140, reproduced by permission from Raven Press Ltd).

straints to the specimen. To be sure that the resultant force and moment at any section of the specimen can be determined, it is then necessary to measure not only the applied loads but the constraining forces and moments set up in reaction to the applied load. Figure 2.11 shows a sketch of a knee specimen being tested in compression at a flexion angle of about 60°. The femur and tibia are attached rigidly to the moving and fixed cross-heads of a materials testing machine which are capable only of translating vertically relative to each other. The apparatus allows only one degree of freedom, that of distraction or interpenetration of the bones. The clamps used to attach the bones to the rig must supply the forces and moments required to suppress flexion, tibial rotation, antero/posterior displacement, etc. The system is statically indeterminate and, unless the forces and moments which constrain motion are measured, the resultant force and moment at the knee is unknown and the test is as likely to reflect the characteristics of the fixation as those of the joint.

Piziali and colleagues, in a series of papers (Piziali *et al.* 1977), described a single degree of freedom apparatus for measuring the stiffness matrix of human knee specimens. It had the important feature that both bones were attached to the platens of the testing machine through six-component force dynamometers so that all the constraining forces and moments were measured and the mechanical state of the specimen could be defined completely. Relative movements of the two bones in any one of the six possible degrees of freedom could be applied and the corresponding constraining forces and moments measured. The difficulty with such an overconstrained system is to ensure that the applied displacements are physiological. It is particularly important, and particularly difficult, to ensure that rotary movements are applied about physiological axes. There are numerous examples of constrained apparatus described in the literature in which the constraining forces and moments were not measured so that the mechanical state of the specimens were not completely defined. In reviewing the literature, a critical reading of apparatus description is necessary to ensure that measurement of constraint has not been overlooked.

2.5 CONCLUSIONS

Measurements of strain in parts of the musculo-skeletal system *in vitro* may be relevant and capable of interpretation only when the resultant force and moment transmitted across the specimen at the site of the measurements is known. Apparatus used to load the specimen may be statically determinate and may require simulation of muscle forces to stabilize the specimen in the presence of known loads. When overconstrained statically indeterminate apparatus is used, the mechanical state of the specimen may not be completely defined unless measurements are made not only of the applied loads but of the constraining reactions as well.

ACKNOWLEDGEMENTS

The design and construction of the rig described in this chapter was supported by a grant from the Arthritis and Rheumatism Council. Drs E. Biden and D. FitzPatrick contributed to the design of the apparatus and the development of the computer programs used to capture and analyse the experimental data. Figures 2.8, 2.9 and 2.10 are reproduced from Dr Biden's thesis.

REFERENCES

Biden, E. (1981) Mechanics of synovial joints. DPhil Thesis, University of Oxford.

Biden, E. and O'Connor, J.J. (1990) Experimental methods used to evaluate knee ligament function, in *Knee Ligaments: Structure, Function, Injury, and Repair, Chapter 8* (eds D.M. Daniel, W.H. Akeson and J.J. O'Connor), Raven Press, New York, pp. 135–52.

Biden, E., O'Connor, J.J. and Goodfellow, J.W. (1984) Tibial rotation in the cadaver knee. *Trans. Orthop. Res. Soc.*, Atlanta, **30**.

Borelli, G.A. (1679) *Di Motu Animalium* (Translation, P. Maquet (1989) Springer-Verlag, Berlin).

Bourne, R.B., Goodfellow, J.W. and O'Connor, J.J. (1978) A functional analysis of various knee arthroplasties. *Trans. Orthop. Res. Soc.*, **24**, 160.

Collins, J.J. (1990) Joint mechanics – modelling the lower limb. DPhil thesis, University of Oxford.

Crandall, S.H., Dahl, N.C. and Lardner, T.J. (1978) *An Introduction to the Mechanics of Solids*, McGraw-Hill, Singapore.

FitzPatrick, D.P. (1989) Mechanics of the knee joint. DPhil thesis, University of Oxford.

Inman, V.T., Ralston, H.J. and Todd, F. (1981) *Human Walking*, Williams and Wilkins, Baltimore.

Kinzel, G.L., Hall, A.S. and Hillberry, B.M. (1972) Measurement of the total motion between two body segments – i. analytical development. *J. Biomech.*, **5**, 93–105.

Maquet, P.G.J. (1976) *Biomechanics of the Knee*, Springer-Verlag, Berlin.

O'Connor, J.J., Shercliff, T., Biden, E. and Goodfellow, J.W. (1989) The geometry of the knee in the sagittal plane. *Proc. I. Mech. E.*, **H203**, 223–33.

O'Connor, J.J., Shercliff, T., FitzPatrick D.P., Biden, E. and Goodfellow, J.W. (1990b) Mechanics of the knee, in *Knee Ligaments: Structure, Function, Injury, and Repair, Chapter 11* (eds D.M. Daniel, W.H. Akeson and J.J. O'Connor), Raven Press, New York, pp. 201–38.

O'Connor, J.J., Shercliff, T., FitzPatrick, D.P., Bradley, J., Daniel, D.M., Biden, E. and Goodfellow, J.W. (1990c) Geometry of the knee, in *Knee Ligaments: Structure, Function, Injury, and Repair, Chapter 10* (eds. D.M. Daniel, W.H. Akeson and J.J. O'Connor), Raven Press, New York, pp. 163–200.

O'Connor, J.J., Biden, E., Bradley, J., FitzPatrick, D.P., Young, S., Kershaw, C., Daniel, D.M. and Goodfellow, J.W. (1990a) The muscle-stabilized knee, in *Knee Ligaments: Structure, Function, Injury, and Repair, Chapter 12* (eds D.M. Daniel, W.H. Akeson and J.J. O'Connor), Raven Press, New York, pp. 239–78.

Paul, J.P. (1967) Forces transmitted by joints in the human body. *Proc. I. Mech. E*, **181** 8–15.

Pauwels, F. (1980) *Biomechanics of the Locomotor Apparatus*, Springer-Verlag, Berlin.

Perry, J., Antonelli, D. and Ford, W. (1975) Analysis of knee-joint forces during flexed-knee stance. *J. Bone Jt. Surg.*, **57A**, 961–7.

Piziali, R.L., Rastegar, J.C. and Nagel, D.A. (1977) Measurement of the non-linear, coupled stiffness characteristics of the human knee. *J. Biomech.*, **10**, 45–51.

Strasser, H. (1917) *Lehrbuch der Muskel-und Gelenkmechanik*, Springer-Verlag, Berlin.

3

Strain gauge measurement

E.G. Little

3.1 INTRODUCTION

Strain gauge model testing is commonly applied in mechanical and civil engineering to complement analytical, numerical and finite element models and to assess the relative behaviour of components. In biomechanics comparative investigation of product performance *in vitro* is often obtained by testing models fitted with different prostheses in a commercial testing machine. Appropriate measures need to be taken to ensure that the data obtained from such tests represents a comparison of the products *in vitro*, as opposed to bias inadvertently introduced into the test by the techniques and procedures used by the experimenter.

In the field of biomechanics, electric resistance strain gauges are used mainly in model testing to provide relative analyses of prostheses (Weightman, 1977), cement mantles (Bushelow and Oh, 1986) and prostheses implanted in cadaveric bone (Finlay *et al.*, 1986). When model testing of this type is carried out, strain gauges may be used not only for strain gauging the model but also for the measurement of forces and couples applied to the model and, in some instances, for the evaluation of the modulus and Poisson's ratio of the materials. It is significant that, in spite of the various applications of strain gauges to model testing in biomechanics, the immense volume of strain measurement literature relating to model testing in traditional mechanical and civil engineering is rarely referenced in the bioengineering journals. Presumably the apparent simplicity of the strain gauge has led to this oversight. Unfortunately the electrical resistance strain gauge is easily misused, resulting in data that either do not reflect the true state of strain at the point being analysed, or that are so significantly biased by intrinsic and extrinsic parameters that the test results do not represent the relative differences deliberately introduced into the model, but rather the relative alteration in experimental technique when changes are made to the model.

It is often not appreciated how easily invalid measurements are obtained. Chalmers (1980) proposed that to obtain accuracy to within 5%, it is necessary to aim for 1%, and that even then 5% is rarely achieved. Perry (1984) implies that 10–15% for quite straightforward work on general engineering components is more commonly achieved, a suggestion which was confirmed by the results of a Society of Experimental Mechanics 'round robin' (Society of Experimental Mechanics Application Committee, 1986). Also, in one of the few articles reporting calibration experiments, Baggott and Lanyon (1977) reported a range of differences between extensiometer and strain gauge readings from +8.8% to −12.6% from tensile tests on brass which is a material with well defined characteristics. While it is commendable that these comparative experiments were carried out, they did not investigate further the reasons for this significant discrepancy. Perry (1984) suggests that the level of accuracy reduces as a function of lack of expertise versus complexity of test, with potentially invalid data being produced from difficult tests carried out by researchers who fail to recognize the expertise required for strain measurement. Only by identifying the parameters that bias the results obtained from strain gauges, such as the more than sixty factors described by Pople (1982a) for a typical installation on a metal product, is it possible to eliminate the sources of error by developing and implementing appropriate codes of practice (British Society for Strain Measurement, 1989) and by conducting fundamental tests to establish the significance of each factor, which may be negligible, or alternatively, if significant, may be compensated for by the application of correction factors (Nickola, 1978). Thus a brief résumé of procedures traditionally applied to model testing for identifying, quantifying, correcting and minimizing errors, together with a brief description of the key factors which prejudice data from strain gauge testing is necessary. Although these factors are drawn from mechanical and civil engineering they have significant relevance to strain gauge model testing in bioengineering.

3.2 PROCEDURES FOR STRAIN GAUGE MODEL TESTING

The parameters influencing the selection of strain gauges: foil, backing material, pattern, grid size, self temperature compensation (STC) number, bridge voltage; and their adhesives, protective coatings, solders and lead wires, are documented (Window and Holister, 1982) and are generally applicable to model testing. In spite of the importance of selecting appropriate materials for strain gauge installations this alone does not guarantee quality results; fundamental tests carried out in parallel with the model test are needed to demonstrate that the strains obtained from an installation are valid. Calibration plays an essential role in assessing the validity of the measurements. Instrument manufacturers normally provide information for calibrating their strain indicators but, according to Pople (1984), it is the experimenter who introduces the most significant errors in the gauging and bridge circuit. Although shunt resistance methods are applied to check the integrity of the complete circuit the results from these tests do not prove that the gauge has been laid up to appropriate standards thereby achieving true strain transmission. For this reason, Pople (1982a) advocated that techniques should be developed to an adequate standard to permit the reproduction of the strain gauge manufacturer's gauge factor. A viable alternative is to carry out a test that provides evidence of the competence of the experimenter, such as the 'user gauge evaluation' test number 62 recommended by the '*Organisation Internationale de Metrologie Legale*'. However, calibration forms only part of the validation procedure.

The principles of dimensional analysis (Durelli *et al.*, 1958) commonly applied in photoelasticity may equally well be applied to strain gauge model testing (Hossdorf, 1974). Although these principles dictate strict geometric similarity between the model and prototype, according to Meyer (1979) it is possible to break the dimensional laws in some instances by applying principles of reduced similarity. However, geometric similarity is essential if the local stresses adjacent to a loaded surface are required, such as in contact and near-field contact problems (Mönch, 1964), which are of importance, for example, in investigations of stresses in cement mantles underlying polyethylene products unsupported by metal plates (Little and O'Keefe, 1989).

Typical parameters for a static model test are given in Table 3.1 and these lead to the dimensionless groups:

$$\Pi_1 = \frac{\sigma}{E} \quad \Pi_2 = \frac{l}{\delta} \quad \Pi_3 = \frac{P}{El^2} \quad \Pi_4 = \epsilon \quad \Pi_5 = \frac{E_1}{E_2} \quad \Pi_6 = \frac{\nu_1}{\nu_2} \quad (3.1)$$

Table 3.1 Typical non-dimensional parameters for a static model test where the basic units are length (L) and force (F) and the physical quantities relating model to prototype are a typical linear dimension (l), moduli of adjacent materials ($E_{1,2}$), Poisson's ratio of adjacent materials ($\nu_{1,2}$), load (P), stress (σ), strain (ϵ) and deflection (δ)

	l	E_1	E_2	ν_1	ν_2	P	σ	ϵ	δ
L	l	−2	−2	0	0	0	−2	0	1
F	0	1	1	0	0	1	1	0	0

When the principles of dimensional analysis are implemented, it is necessary to model the ratio of moduli between adjacent sections. However, modulus matching is difficult to achieve, and although it may appear an attractive proposition to obtain a suitable modulus by including fillers to modify the properties of epoxy systems, difficulties emerge in controlling the degree of settlement leading to variations in characteristics within the section. Furthermore, considerable addition of filler often makes the mix highly viscous leading to air entrapment. Exothermic reactions may be induced by adding accelerators to cold curing epoxy. Finally Müller (1971) has described the variation in properties as a function of cure time. Extensive mechanical testing is thus needed to ascertain the mechanical properties of different epoxy systems (Riegner and Scotese, 1971). Low modulus plastics offer advantages for modelling the limited range of moduli encountered in biomechanical investigations, but because considerable variations often arise in the properties reported in manufacturers' data sheets, laboratory testing is desirable. Considerable technical difficulties may emerge here when strain gauges are employed.

From the dimensionless group, Π_6, formed above it can be inferred that even if the ratio of moduli are correctly modelled, errors may be induced by mismatch of Poisson's ratio. General effects of the influence of Poisson's ratio are discussed by Stansfield (1965) and the bias evaluated relevant to contact problems (Pao *et al.*, 1971; Macmillan, 1989), to multiconnected bodies (Frocht, 1948; Timoshenko and Goodier, 1951), to three-dimensional analyses (Fessler and Lewin, 1960) and to composite materials (Jones, 1975). Calculations are recommended to determine the prejudice caused by this mismatch (Mönch, 1964), but in biomechanical investigations applicable theoretical models seldom exist.

The dimensional groups in equation (3.1) are for materials which are isotropic and homogeneous and therefore not representative of bone. Gross distortions are present when these materials are applied to modelling anisotropic situations as in the model test of Little and O'Keefe (1989) shown in Figure 3.1 which attempts to simulate *in vitro* the stress at selected sites in the cement mantle underlying the tibial component of the Geomedic knee prosthesis. However, despite these limitations, this model test produced non-linear results, representing a fractured interface between the materials modelling the cement–bone interface, and stresses in the anterior–posterior direction indicative of tibial component tilting (Little, 1990). To obtain useful data from models with defined mechanical properties the results may be compared with data from finite element studies (Little, 1985a). Once similar trends are obtained from both techniques, an enhanced understanding of the merits and limitations of each procedure emerges, leading to a better informed engineering judgement; moreover, once acceptable correlations have been obtained, the material properties may be updated in the finite element work to model the anisotropic situation.

The mechanical properties of metals, such as modulus and Poisson's ratio, are frequently measured with electrical resistance strain gauges; however, incorrect data are obtained, and may go unrecognized, if strain gauges are used for these measurements on plastics and composites since heating (Little, 1982) and reinforcement (Little *et al.*, 1990) can induce significant errors in the measurement of strain. Creep or relaxation moduli are more appropriate than tensile test data for plastic model studies (Nickola, 1978; Little, 1985a, b), but the measurement of strain in these tests ideally requires precision, special-purpose machines (Dunn *et al.*, 1964; Thomas, 1969; Thomas and Turner, 1969) and suitably calibrated extensiometry (Benham and McCammond, 1971). Furthermore, to avoid measuring the transformed reduced stiffness term (Pagano and Halpin, 1968), bow-tie specimens (Jones, 1975) are necessary for the evaluation of the properties of composite materials, and the limitations of rail shear tests (ASTM, D 4255–82) applied to measure shear moduli should be recognized (Whitney *et al.*, 1971). Mismatch between the thermal expansion of the material and the STC number of the strain gauge can cause gross errors in measurements taken on plastic and composite materials, so that compensation procedures are essential (Mitchell, 1979).

Selecting the site for mounting the gauges on the model requires considerable expertise; for example, Marsh (1989) observed that the failure to implement established procedures in fatigue testing of prototype structures can result in crack initiation at sites remote from the areas covered with strain gauges. In biomechanics strain gauges too often appear to be mounted on models in random positions. The use of brittle lacquer (Macduff, 1978), photoelastic coatings, finite element studies (Society of Automotive Engineers, 1988) or an examination of fractured components can all provide information to assist in the identification of relevant sites. However, brittle lacquer fractures perpendicular to the maximum principal strain (Cunningham and Yovorsky, 1957; Greszczuk, 1965; Chaturvedi and Agarwal, 1978) and photoelastic coatings indicate maximum in-plane shearing strain (Kenward and Hindle, 1970) but not necessarily the maximum shearing strain and for composite materials these strains are not necessarily coincident with maximum principal stress and maximum in-plane shearing stress. Furthermore, finite element studies should be accompanied by results from appropriate bench mark tests (Hitchens, 1987; Hitchens *et al.*, 1987). In the analysis reported by Little *et al.* (1985) the approach adopted is appropriate, but recent bench mark tests show that the finite-element data reported therein are incorrect.

Strain gradients pose a further problem; if subject to gradients, the

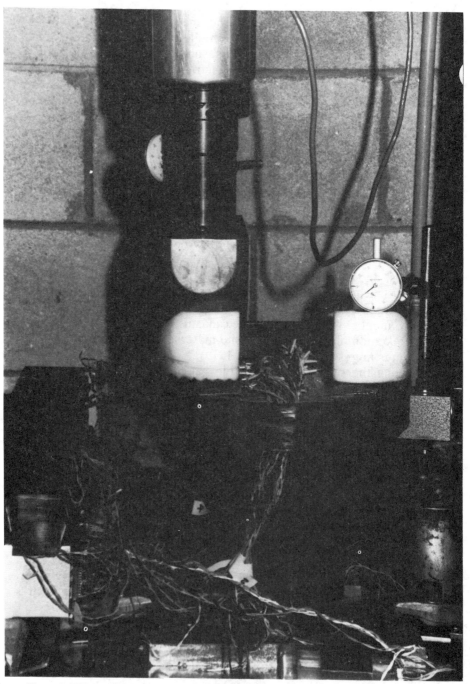

Figure 3.1 Three-dimensional embedded strain gauge analysis of the cement mantle underlying the tibial plateau of the Geomedic knee prosthesis.

grid of the strain gauge integrates the strain and indicates strains that are completely unrepresentative of the true strain at a point. A classic example cited by Perry (1984) shows how a gauge mounted adjacent to a hole in a plate subjected to tension induces an error in excess of 20% when the grid of length and width is equal to 0.2 of the radius of the hole. Pople (1980) found that mistakes were induced by the combination of gradients and errors in axial positioning; however, miniature gauges suitably positioned and orientated overcame this problem. It is suggested here that where strain concentrations require evaluation, the data from miniature gauges mounted onto large scale models, designed in accordance with the dimensional laws discussed above, should be analysed by appropriate techniques (Dhillon and Thompson, 1988; Thompson and Brodland, 1988); alternatively, photoelastic methods may be applied.

Serious errors are induced by strain gauge misalignment. To illustrate this point Pople (1980) considered the measurement of thrust on a shaft subjected to a torque-to-thrust ratio of 7.5:1; one degree of gauge misalignment with the shaft axis led to an error of 53% in the measurement of thrust. Errors such as these are reduced by implementing gauge lay-up procedures using microscopes with cross-wires, which are commonly used in transducer applications and have potential for laboratory model testing. Alternatively, photographic techniques may quantify successfully gauge misalignment errors, leading to the application of correction factors (Pople, 1982b). Further details of the influence of gauge misalignment are reported for single and rectangular rosettes (Perry, 1969) with errors being very significant in orthotropic composites (Tuttle and Brinson, 1984).

Once the site for mounting the gauge is established and the orientation determined, mistakes are induced by inaccurate gauge positioning. The data reported by Little *et al.* (1990) show how a systematic error of 2% can result from a deviation of only 0.05 mm in embedding a strain gauge at a distance of 2.55 mm from the neutral axis in a cantilever bend test. The statistical procedures advocated by Meyer (1979) and Coleman and Steel (1989) and applied in this case may be used to indicate the prejudice created by each parameter. The most important parameters biasing the data are thus recognized, and compensation is made possible.

The unsuitable selection of power density for gauges mounted onto or embedded into plastics and composites having poor thermal conductivity can lead to excessive local heating reducing the modulus of the underlying material with resulting changes in strain transmission and measurement of apparent strain (Nickola, 1978). In these situations continuous voltage supplies can be utilized providing that results from fundamental tests indicate that a suitable selection of gauge grid area, gauge resistance, gauge backing material, bridge voltage, gauge circuit and sectional model thickness produce reliable data (Little, 1982). Pulsed systems, employed by various researchers (Bray and Desogus, 1970; Mitchell, 1979; MaCalvey, 1982) required fundamental testing leading to the selection of suitable pulse amplitudes, pulse durations and frequencies which are dependent upon the application.

The strain gauge manufacturer provides a gauge factor which is established under ideal conditions (Pople, 1982a); when the gauge is applied to materials or is used in environments other than those under which it was calibrated changes in characteristics occur. Strain gauge applications on plastics and composites produce variations in gauge factor which depend upon the modulus and sectional thickness of the model material, gauge backing (Swan, 1973; Kelly, 1974; Mitchell, 1979), the gauge pattern, gauge length, solder buds and lead wires (Mitchell, 1979), strain field (Kelly, 1974; Mitchell, 1979), power density (Lawton, 1968) and thickness of the protective coating. In composite materials the gauge factor may differ directionally (Perry, 1985a), with each grid being affected to a dissimiliar extent. In these circumstances compensation is achieved via a suitable calibration procedure (Mitchell, 1979; Perry, 1985b, 1986). Failure to implement such a procedure can result in data that cannot be converted to principal strains and are not simply related in sections of differing thickness.

Invalid data may also be obtained from models subject to incorrect boundary conditions. Typically, contact stress problems are analysed using either analytical (Johnson, 1985) or finite-element procedures either neglecting friction (Bartel *et al.*, 1986) or incorporating friction (Pascoe and Mottershead, 1988, 1989). The results from these complex investigations require experimental validation from model tests which produce realistic load transfer between mating components, achieved only by satisfying the dimensional laws of strict geometric similarity between the mating components (Mönch, 1964). In these situations, stresses may depend upon the geometry of contact (Frocht, 1948), the moduli ratio of the surfaces in contact (Bray, 1981), Poisson's ratio as discussed previously, the thickness of the layers and whether they are bonded or unbonded (Pao *et al.*, 1971), the coefficients of friction (Bray, 1981) and the surface finish between the contacting bodies. These examples illustrate the point expressed by Heywood (1969) that the often quoted St Venant's principle is very crude. The necessity of obtaining appropriate contact conditions between mating components and ascertaining their effects upon load transmission in tibial plateaux (Chao *et al.*, 1977; Little *et al.*, 1985) and acetabular cups (Rapperport *et al.*, 1985, 1987) appear to have been recognized by only a few investigators in biomechanics. Sliding and rolling contact problems investigated by embedded strain gauge methods (Bazergui and Meyer,

1968; Derenne and Bazergui, 1971; Berme *et al.*, 1975) have not yet been related to analyses of implants.

The simulation of fixed and simply supported edges presents its own special problems; as Hossdorf (1974) points out, both encastré fixation and simple edge supports are easily formulated analytically, but never achieved perfectly in practice. Unless contact conditions are of importance, measurements at and close to fixation sites and supports are best avoided. The acceptable distance from the boundary at which measurements are valid is application-dependent and requires investigation in each case.

Methods employed in metrology laboratories (Bray *et al.*, 1990) for analysis of forces and couples during the design and calibration of multicomponent balances are also applicable to model testing. These methods include the use of lever and wire pulley arrangements (Dubois, 1974), with pulleys supported on small diameter bearings or knife edges (Figure 3.2), thus minimizing friction, and wires aligned with cathotometers. Load transmission from the loading apparatus to the model is generally via a sphere resting in a conical seating (Figure 3.2), crossed knife edge rocker bearings (Bray, 1981) shown under assessment in Figure 3.3 or a sphere lapped onto a spherical seating (Debham and Jenkins, 1972). Rolling bearings are avoided since frictional effects produce variable data depending on the direction of the load application (Hossdorf, 1974) and although hydraulic control systems have advantages for producing simultaneous application of force components, drifting and instability can occur. Devices to provide protection from overloading to prevent damage during testing are advisable.

Commercial testing machines have been found to apply, in some situations, significant forces and couples other than that of the axial load. For example, Little (1990) obtained different data from compression tests on the prismatic bar shown in Figure 3.3 depending upon the angular orientation of the bar about its vertical axis, when subjected to loading via an established procedure (Debham and Jenkins, 1976). The amplitude of the sine waves was influenced by a lack of parallelism in the platens, loading jig and bar end faces, together with minor errors in perpendicularity between the bar axis and end faces, frame backlash, gauge positioning and gauge orientation. Elsewhere, models set in testing apparatus and loading to induce restrained bending produced parasitic forces and couples causing distortion of the machine frame (Rossetto *et al.*, 1975). These adverse effects are present in the investigations reported by Little (1985a) and Little and O'Keefe (1989) and further research to quantify them is in progress. Special loading frames similar to that shown in Figure 3.2, albeit expensive to make and set up, have advantages for critical tests (Smith, 1977). However, if such

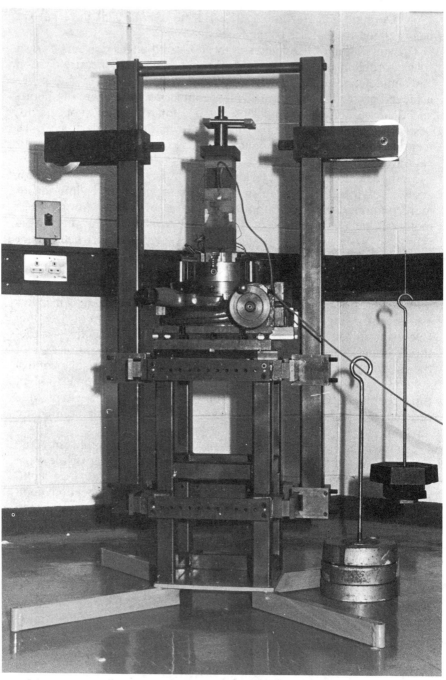

Figure 3.2 Frame for multicomponent balance calibration.

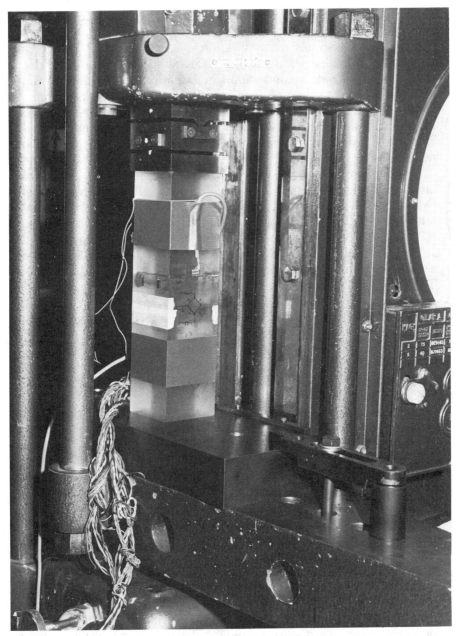

Figure 3.3 Compression test on a prismatic bar containing embedded three-dimensional strain rosettes. The load is transmitted to the bar through crossed knife edge rocker bearings.

apparatus is inadequately designed, deflections will produce unacceptable misalignment of the applied forces.

Figure 3.4 illustrates an application of these principles where an hemipelvis is loaded via a floating frame supported on a long wire, thus eliminating side loading, and simulation of muscle forces with a wire-pulley-deadweight arrangement. However, in the arrangement shown, the methods used to join the wires to the pelvis do not represent ideal muscle attachment and the sacro-iliac joint is inadequately modelled, thus indicating the limitations associated with model testing in this situation.

Commercial testing apparatus is used in displacement control if either relaxation moduli or compensation procedures are implemented (Meyer, 1979) or in load control if creep data are available. In the latter case the maximum load is applied initially to the model which is then unloaded and allowed to relax followed by preloading and subsequent loading in increasing increments, thus avoiding errors associated with creep recovery of viscoelastic materials (Thomas and Turner, 1969). Data obtained from single load increments are statistically unsound. Incremental loading procedures require sensible implementation (Smith, 1976) but have an added advantage in that they allow regression techniques to be applied.

Strain gauge model testing of civil engineering structures is accompanied by carefully chosen check measurements and/or by measurement of forces and couples (Hossdorf, 1974). Multicomponent shear element balances originally designed by Boyle (1970) and used by Molland (1976) for wind tunnel applications, may be applied in model testing but require calibration. Alternative designs of balances may also be applicable.

Repeatable measurements are achievable even in an unsatisfactory test; therefore, to ensure that strains purporting to be representative of differences between products are not simply the results of variations in the experimental procedure, reproducibility testing is necessary. This entails dismantling the entire rig, reassembling it and retesting at incremental loadings. The residual variance about the regression line may be estimated or a quicker procedure is to calculate the variance from reproducibility tests at a single load level. Models fitted with dowels and tenons form a reliable method of providing repeatable and reproducible alignment in the same test apparatus, but do not guarantee that other relevant features, such as variable contact resistance between connectors due to reassembly, have been replicated; neither do they ensure that the strains recorded from the model are accurate.

If all the factors described above are taken into account and correction factors are applied together with compensation for changes in gauge factor, STC mismatch, transverse sensitivity, lead wire desensiti-

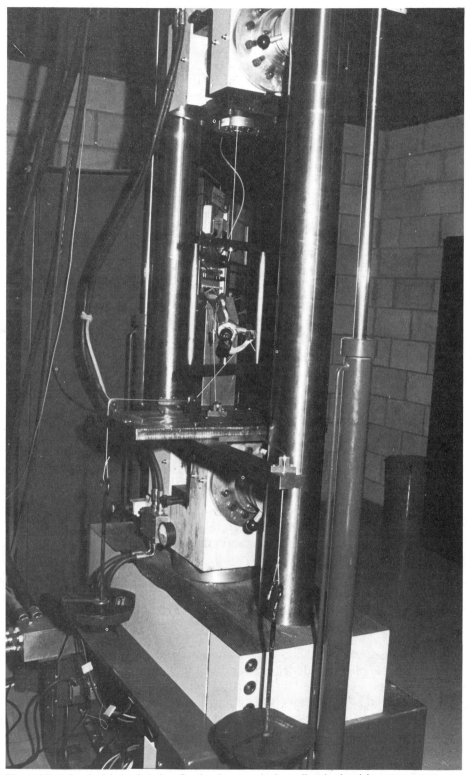

Figure 3.4 A hemipelvis loaded via a floating frame and wire pulley dead weight arrangement.

zation etc. (Pople, 1979), gross errors may still be made in converting from strain to stress owing to the failure to appreciate that the relationship $E = \sigma/\epsilon$ is not generally applicable. Even in a tensile test, an analysis of stress and strain at a point demonstrates the possibility of the presence of (1) strains of opposite sign to the stress, (2) strain in the absence of stress and (3) stress without strain, depending upon the plane examined.

Two-element rectangular rosettes are suitable for measuring principal strain if located in the principal strain directions, which are usually identified by brittle lacquer or photoelastic coating studies prior to installing the strain gauges, and which may not be coincident with principal stresses in composites. In the absence of information indicating the principal strain directions, a three-element rosette is required. The relevant constitutive relations for isotropic and orthotropic materials are described by Jones (1975). All of the constitutive relations require the material constants, and any exposure to analysis of composites will have convinced the investigator that these quantities are difficult to measure.

Thus, investigations which purport to provide a relative evaluation of products may in fact provide nothing more than a relative evaluation of the alterations in the testing procedure when changes are made to the models under test. If this is to be avoided, meticulous investigations must be carried out to relevant standards. The UK National Measurement Accreditation Service (NAMAS) currently provides accreditation to laboratories which satisfy the appropriate standards required for calibration and commercial testing. Agreement is emerging between certain states of the EC on mutual recognition for such accreditation (Chalmers, 1989), unfortunately the NAMAS recommendations for strain gauge measurement are still in draft form, mainly because the many varied applications of the electric resistance strain gauge makes agreement upon measurement standards difficult to achieve. The form of the recommendations in preparation are as yet unknown and the long term implications for strain gauge model testing in biomechanics unclear.

3.3 CONCLUSIONS

When electrical resistance gauges are used in model testing, test variables are application dependent and will vary according to techniques and procedures applied in a particular laboratory. Only by investigation of the parameters which may potentially bias the data can corrective methods be applied. What may appear to the uninformed as secondary effects must not be overlooked, since the failure to recognize the existence of these factors and the complexity of their interrelationships can lead to the misinterpretation of test results and the reporting of erroneous information.

ACKNOWLEDGEMENTS

The author wishes to thank Howmedica International Inc. for funding the work described in this chapter and colleagues within BSSM for their helpful criticism of the model testing carried out in his laboratory: Bob Boyle (Concepts (Laleham)), Ray Jenkins (NPL), Jim MacKinnon (NEL), John Pople (Vickers) and Geoff Chalmers (Measurements Group Inc.).

REFERENCES

Baggott, D.G. and Lanyon, L.E. (1977) An independent post mortem calibration of electrical resistance strain gauges bonded to bone surfaces *in vivo*. *J. Biomech.*, **10**, 615–22.

Bartel, D.L., Bicknell, V.L., Ithaca, M.S., and Wright, T.M. (1986) The effect of conformity, thickness and material on stresses in ultra-high molecular weight components for total hip replacement. *J. Bone Jt. Surg*, **68–A**, 1041–51.

Bazergui, A. and Meyer, M.L. (1968) Embedded strain gauges for the measurement of strains in rolling contact. *Exptl. Mech.*, **8**, 433–41.

Benham, P.P. and McCammond, D. (1971) Studies of creep contraction ratio in thermoplastics. *Plast. Polym.*, **39**, 130–6.

Berme, N., Mengi, Y. and Tarhan, A. (1975) The effect of sliding load on strain gauges embedded under the contact surface. *Strain*, **11** (4), 169–72.

Boyle, H.B. (1970) The strain gauge: an aid to the development of marine transport. *Strain*, **6** (4), 151–5.

Bray, A. (1981) The role of stress analysis in the design of force standard transducers. *Exptl. Mech.*, **21** (1), 1–20.

Bray, A., Barbato, G. and Levi, R. (1990) *Theory and Practice of Force Measurement*, Academic Press, London.

Bray, A. and Desogus, S. (1970) Gli estensimetri annegati: nuovo metodo per l'analisi tridimensionale delle tensioni. *Ingegneria Meccanica*, **19** (12), 29–36.

British Society for Strain Measurement (1989) *Code of Practice for the Installation of Electrical Resistance Strain Gauges*, BSSM, Newcastle upon Tyne.

Bushelow, M. and Oh, I. (1986) The effect of acetabular cup polyethylene thickness upon cement mantle strain: an *in vitro* strain gauge study. *11th Annual Meeting of Society of Biomaterials*, San Diego, p. 124.

Chalmers, G. (1980) The dangers of the 5% mentality. BSSM and I. Prod. Engng. Annual Conf.: Product Liability and Reliability, Aston.

Chalmers, G. (1989) Europe 1992 – standards, testing and certification. *Strain*, **25** (2), 47–50.

Chao, E.Y.S., Wong, H.W., Frain, W.E. and Coventry, M.B. (1977) Stress analysis of the Geometric knee under static loading. *ASME Appl. Mech. Fluid Mech. Bio. Engng. Conf.*, New Haven, CT, paper no. 77.

Chaturvedi, S.K. and Agarwal, B.D. (1978) Brittle coating studies on fibrous composites. *Strain*, **14** (4), 131–6.

Coleman, H.W. and Steel, W.G. (1989) *Experimentation and Uncertainty Analysis for Engineers*, John Wiley, New York.

Cunningham, J.H. and Yovorsky, J.M. (1957) The brittle lacquer technique of stress analysis as applied to anisotropic materials. *SESA Proc.*, **XIV**, 101–8.

Debham, R.C. and Jenkins, R.F. (1972) The influence of end loading conditions on the performance of strain gauge load cells. *VDI-Berichte*, **176**, 53–60.

Debham, R.C. and Jenkins, R.F. (1976) Sources of measurement error during an intercomparison of force standard machines. *Proc. Round Table Discussion on Measurement of Force and Mass, 7th IMEKO Congress*, London, pp. 18–39.

Derenne, M. and Bazergui, A. (1971) Advances in the embedded strain gauge technique with an application to contact problems. *Exptl. Mech.*, **11**, 105–12.

Dhillon, S.S. and Thompson, J.C. (1988) A simplified method for predicting stress concentration in notches from experimental stress data. *Strain*, **24** (3), 95–8.

Dubois, M. (1974) Design and manufacture of high precision strain gauge dynamometers and balance at the ONERA Modane centre. *Strain*, **10** (4), 188–94.

Dunn, C.M.R., Mills, W.H. and Turner, S. (1964) Creep in thermoplastics – review of apparatus for creep measurements. *Brit. Plast.*, 386–92.

Durelli, A.J., Phillips, A.E. and Tsao, C.H. (1958) Dimensional analysis, in *Introduction to the Theoretical and Experimental Analysis of Stress and Strain*, McGraw-Hill, New York, pp. 278–302.

Fessler, H. and Lewin, B.H. (1960) A study of large strain and the effect of different values of Poisson's ratio, *Brit. J. Appl. Phys.*, **11**, 273–7.

Finlay, J.B., Bourne, R., Landsberg, R. and Andreae, P. (1986) Pelvic stresses *in vitro*–1 malsizing of the endoprotheses. *J. Biomech.*, **19** (9), 703–14.

Frocht, M.M. (1948) *Photoelasticity, Vol II*, John Wiley, New York.

Greszczuk, L.B. (1965) Effect of material orthotropy on the directions of principal stresses and strains, in *Orientation Effects in the Mechanical Behaviour of Anistropic Structural Materials*, ASTM STP no. 405.

Heywood, R.B. (1969) *Photoelasticity for Designers*, Pergamon Press, Oxford.

Hitchens, D. (1987) *Linear Static Bench Marks, Vol. 2*, NAFEMS Publications, NEL, Glasgow.

Hitchens, D., Kamoulakos, A. and Davies, G.A.O. (1987) *Linear Static Bench Marks, Vol. 1*, NAFEMS Publications, NEL. Glasgow.

Hossdorf, H. (1974) *Model Analysis of Structures*, Van Nostrand Reinhold, Wokingham.

Johnson, K.L. (1985) *Contact Mechanics*, Cambridge University Press, Cambridge.

Jones, R.M. (1975) *Mechanics of Composite Materials*, Hemisphere, New York.

Kelly, P.D. (1974) Strain gauge reinforcement and plastic relaxation effects in the analysis of ABS plastic parts. *SPE Ann. Tech. Conf.*, San Francisco, pp. 305–7.

Kenward, K.T. and Hindle, G.R. (1970) Analysis of strain in fibre-reinforced materials. *J. Strain Anal.*, **5** (4), 309–15.

Lawton, B. (1968) The use of plastic models to evaluate thermal strains in diesel engine pistons. *J. Strain Anal.*, **3** (3), 176–86.

Little, E.G. (1982) Effects of self heating when using a continuous bridge voltage for strain gauging epoxy models. *Strain*, **18**, 131–4.

Little, E.G. (1985a) Experimental stress analysis of the Geomedic knee joint using embedded strain gauges. *Engng. Med.,* **14** (2), 69–74.

Little, E.G. (1985b) Compressive creep behaviour of irradiated ultra high molecular weight polyethylene at 37°C. *Engng. Med.,* **14** (2), 85–7.

Little, E.G. (1990) Three dimensional strain rosettes from an analysis of the Geomedic knee prosthesis and underlying cement fixation, in *Applied Stress Analysis* (eds T.E. Hyde and E. Ollerton), Elsevier, Barking.

Little, E.G., Kneafsey, A.G., Lynch, P. and Kennedy, M. (1985) The design of a model for a three dimensional stress analysis of the cement layer beneath the medial plateau of a knee prosthesis. *J. Biomech.,* **18** (2), 157–60.

Little, E.G. and O'Keefe, D. (1989) An experimental technique for the investigation of three dimensional stress in bone cement underlying a tibial plateau. *Proc. I. Mech. E.,* **203 H1**, 35–41.

Little, E.G., Tocher, D. and O'Donnell, P. (1990) Strain gauge reinforcement of plastics. *Strain,* **26** (3), 91–8.

MaCalvey, L.F. (1982) Strain measurement on low modulus materials. *BSSM Annual Conference, State of the Art in Measurement Techniques,* University of Surrey, Guildford.

Macduff, I.B. (1978) Brittle lacquer technique, in *Methods and Practice for Stress and Strain Measurement Part 3: Optical Methods for Determining Strain and Displacement,* BSSM Monograph, Newcastle upon Tyne.

Macmillan, N.H. (1989) The influence of Poisson's ratio on Hertzian contact stresses. *J. Mater. Sci. Let.,* **8**, 340–2.

Marsh, K.J. (1989) The role of measurement in fatigue design assessment. *Strain,* **25** (4), 127–33.

Meyer, M.L. (1979) *Structural Model Testing in Methods and Practice for Stress and Strain Measurement – Part 4: Selection and Application of Experimental Method,* BSSM monograph, Newcastle upon Tyne.

Mitchell, D. (1979) Strain and temperature measurements on epoxy resin models. *Transducer Technol.,* **1** (4), 21–5.

Molland, A.F. (1976) *The Design, Construction and Calibration of a Five Component Strain Gauge Wind Tunnel Dynamometer,* Ship Science report 1/77, University of Southampton.

Mönch, E. (1964) Similarity and model laws in photoelastic experiments. *Exptl. Mech.,* **4**, 141–50.

Müller, R.K. (1971) *Handbuch der Modellstatik,* Springer-Verlag, Heidelburg.

Nickola, W.E. (1978) Strain gauge measurement on plastic models. *BSSM Ann. Conf.: Applications of Materials Testing to Experimental Stress Analysis,* Bradford.

Pagano, N.J. and Halpin, J.C. (1968) Influence of end constraint in the testing of anisotropic bodies. *J. Comp. Mater.,* **2**, 18–31.

Pao, Y.C., Wu, T.S. and Chiu, Y.P. (1971) Bounds on the maximum contact stress of an indented elastic layer. *J. Appl. Mech.,* **38**, 608–14.

Pascoe, S.K. and Mottershead, J.E. (1988) Linear elastic contact problems using curved elements and including dynamic friction. *Int. J. Num. Methods Engng.* **26**, 1631–43.

Pascoe, S.K. and Mottershead, J.E. (1989) Two new finite element contact algorithms. *Comput. Struct.,* **32** (1), 137–44.

Perry, C.C. (1969) Strain gauge misalignment errors. *Instrum. Control Syst.*, **42**, 137–9.

Perry, C.C. (1984) The electric resistance strain gauge revisited. *Exptl. Mech.*, **24** (4), 286–99.

Perry, C.C. (1985a) Experimental stress analysis of reinforced plastics. 40th Int. Conf. Reinforced Plastics, Composites Institute, Session 5–C, 1–7.

Perry, C.C. (1985b) Strain gauge reinforcement on low modulus materials. *Exptl. Tech.*, **9** (5), 25–7.

Perry, C.C. (1986) Strain gauge reinforcement on orthotropic materials. *Exptl. Tech.*, **10** (2), 20–4.

Pople, J. (1979) *BSSM Strain Measurement Reference Book*, BSSM, Newcastle upon Tyne.

Pople, J. (1980) DIY strain gauge transducers. *Strain*, **16** (1), 23–36.

Pople, J. (1982a) Errors and uncertainties in strain measurement, in *Strain Gauge Technology* (eds A.L. Window and G.S. Holister), Applied Science Publishers, Barking.

Pople, J. (1982b) Gauge installation and protection in hostile environments, in *Strain Gauge Technology* (eds A.L. Window and G.S. Holister), Applied Science Publishers, Barking, 209–64.

Pople, J. (1984) Errors in strain measurement – the human factor (or how much do I contribute?). *Exptl. Tech.*, **8** (9), 34–8.

Rapperport, D.J., Carter, D.R. and Schurman, D.J. (1985) Contact finite element stress analysis of the hip joint. *J. Orthop. Res.*, **3**, 435–46.

Rapperport, D.J., Carter, D.R. and Schurman, D.J. (1987) Contact finite element stress analysis of porous ingrowth, acetabular cup implantation, ingrowth and loosening. *J. Orthop. Res.*, **5**, 548–61.

Riegner, E.I. and Scotese, A.E. (1971) Aluminium reinforced epoxy models. *Exptl. Mech.*, **11**, 38–45.

Rossetto, S., Bray, A. and Levi, R. (1975) Three-dimensional strain rosettes: pattern selection and performance evaluation. *Exptl. Mech.*, **15** (10), 375–81.

Smith, J.D. (1976) Misuse of regression techniques in calibration. *Strain*, **13** (4), 120–1.

Smith, J.D. (1977) Practical problems in calibration of torque tubes. *Strain*, **14** (4), 148–51.

Society of Automotive Engineers (1988) *Fatigue Design Handbook*, 2nd edn., SAE, Pennsylvania.

Society of Experimental Mechanics Applications Committee (1986) SEM strain gauge round robin. *Exptl. Tech.*, **10** (9), 27–31.

Stanssfield, F.M. (1965) Some notes on the use of perspex models for the investigation of machine tool structures. *Proc. 6th Int. Conf. Machine Tool Design and Research*, Manchester.

Swan, J.W. (1973) Resistance strain gauges on thermoplastics. *Strain*, **9** (2), 56–9.

Thomas, D.A. (1969) Uniaxial compressive creep studies. *Plast. Polym.*, **37**, 485–91.

Thomas, D.A. and Turner, S. (1969) Experimental technique in uniaxial tensile creep testing, in *Testing of Polymers, Vol. 4* (ed. W.E. Brown), Interscience, New York.

Thompson, J.C. and Brodland, G.W. (1988) Analysis of strain averaged data from finite length gauges and predictions of peak strain for planar notch and fillet problems. *Strain*, **24** (4), 147–52.

Timoshenko, S. and Goodier, J.N. (1951) *Theory of Elasticity*, McGraw-Hill, New York.

Tuttle, M.E. and Brinson, H.F. (1984) Resistance foil strain gauge technology as applied to composite materials. *Exptl. Mech.*, **24**, 54–65.

Weightman, B. (1977) Stress analysis, in *The Scientific Basis of Joint Replacement* (eds S.A.V. Swanson and M.A.R. Freeman), Pitman, Tonbridge Wells.

Whitney, J.M., Stansbarger, D.L. and Howell, H.B. (1971) Analysis of the rail shear test – applications and limitations. *J. Comp. Mater.*, **5**, 24–34.

Window, A.L. and Holister, G.S. (eds) (1982) *Strain Gauge Technology*, Applied Science Publishers, Barking.

4

In vitro strain measurement in bone

M. Dabestani

4.1 INTRODUCTION

The initial *in vitro* measurement of the mechanical properties of bone was by Wertheim (1847) and since then a variety of techniques and analytical procedures have been developed and applied. These techniques include non-destructive methods such as ultrasound, (Abenschein and Hyatt, 1970), holographic interferometry (Manley *et al.*, 1987), photoelastic analysis (Milch, 1940), and the use of semiconductor (Bonfield *et al.*, 1973) and resistance strain gauges (Bonfield and O'Connor, 1978) on whole bones or on specimens of bone in either destructive or non-destructive tests. While each of these methods are suitable in their own right the objective is to obtain a testing procedure that can fulfil the experimental requirements. The maintenance of the moisture state, temperature, applied stress, strain rate and the identification of the anisotropic properties control the strain measurement technique in bone *in vitro*. For example, in the case of ultrasound the testing frequency is considerably higher than the physiological loading rates. Any strain measuring device should be capable of accommodating the physiological requirements of bone and the effectiveness of the measuring system in terms of its sensitivity, capability and versatility is important for the accurate measurement of strain in bone.

The suitability of a variety of strain gauge devices for application to bone has been examined by comparative studies *in vitro*; the Tuckerman Optical Gauge agreed with capacitance gauges within 5% (Bonfield *et al.*, 1973) and with electrical resistance strain gauges within 10% (Bonfield and Clark, 1973). Wright and Hayes (1979) tested electrical resistance strain gauges versus extensometry versus total displacement measurement. They obtained good agreement between strain gauge and extensometer, but the total displacement measurement resulted in large errors. *In vivo*, Baggott and Lanyon (1977) calibrated electrical resistance strain gauges versus mirror extensometers. The latter are sensitive for strains greater than 10^{-5}, while the former offer 10^{-6} sensitivity.

Apart from providing a more sensitive direct measurement of strain, electrical resistance strain gauges offer advantages; the specimen can be immersed in physiological saline and tested within a wide temperature range, for dynamic testing they provide a continuous and simultaneous direct measurement of strain and choice of signal processing, analogue or digital which in turn provides flexibility of analysis. However, it must be noted that because strain gauges only provide point information, the areas of interest must be identified prior to the application of the gauge.

4.2 BONE PRESERVATION AND PREPARATIONS

As in all biological systems, the *in vitro* experiment cannot fully mimic the *in vivo* environment, therefore it is necessary to consider whether the data obtained from *in vitro* studies are representative of the *in vivo* behaviour. Evans (1973), reviewed the work of many previous workers including Gurdjian and Lissner (1945), Stevens and Ray (1962), Lissner and Roberts (1966) and Greenberg *et al.* (1968), and concluded that the differences in mechanical properties and biochemical behaviour of living and dead bone, when tested under similar conditions, are insignificant. Dempster and Liddicoat (1952) found that dry bone shows a significant degree of brittleness compared with wet bone, therefore it is important that bone is not dehydrated during testing. Seldin and Hirsch (1966) and Currey (1988) suggested that bone is unaffected by slow drying provided it is thoroughly re-wetted before testing. Evans (1973) confirmed that while freezing does not alter the mechanical properties of bone, freeze-drying has irreversible effects on its microstructure (Pelker *et al.*, 1984). Thus results from experiments with dead bone in fresh and moist condition are valid for extrapolation and comparable with the living animal.

Specimen preparation, that is cutting and machining, should be carried out with continuous water irrigation or under water to prevent the specimen drying out and to reduce thermal damage. Bone should be stored at $-20°C$, defrosted at room temperature and tested while immersed in a physiological saline, for example Ringer's solution. The preparation of bone specimens is straightforward. The bone is thawed, cleaned, the periosteum removed with a scalpel and coarse grit diamond paper, the ends sawn off and the marrow removed, resulting in a hollow cylinder of compact bone from which specimens can be machined to any desired size or shape. Any regions containing large periosteal blood vessels are discarded. In the case of whole bone preparation for strain gauge application the major concerns are the regions containing periosteal blood vessels, and the areas where the cortical bone is extremely thin. These areas must be sealed and prepared before the application of the strain gauges (Finlay *et al.*, 1982). The region is air dried, a thin layer of catalyst (e.g. 200-catalyst, Micromeasurements) is applied and after drying for 1 min two drops of methyl–2–cyanoacrylate (M Bond 200, Micromeasurements) are applied to the area and pressed into a thin layer using finger pressure and a piece of polyethylene sheet. After 1 min the pressure is removed and the area allowed to harden for a further 5 min before the area is smoothed down with No. 400 silicon-carbide paper.

4.3 ATTACHMENT OF STRAIN GAUGES

The operation of strain gauges is based on the strain sensitivity of an electrically conductive material. Strain sensitivity is defined as the ratio of the relative change in electrical resistance of a conductor to the relative change in its length, i.e. it is a function of the dimensional changes, elongation and cross-sectional contraction, which occur when a conductor is stretched, plus any changes in the basic resistivity of the material with strain. When the conductor is stretched, for an extension Δl, there will be an associated reduction in the cross-section area $(\nu\Delta l)^2$ due to Poisson's ratio effects. These combine and result in an increase in the resistance of the conductor.

If a gauge is bonded to a test material with a different coefficient of thermal expansion than that of the gauge material, a change in temperature will produce strain in the gauge and hence, a resistance change due to the difference in expansion. This strain is referred to as temperature induced 'apparent-strain', and is one of the most serious potential sources of error. Most modern resistance strain gauges are self-temperature compensated type, which principally consist of copper–nickel and modified nickel–chromium that have been processed to adjust the basic temperature coefficient of resistance to compensate for the resistance change due to differential expansion effects for various materials (Chalmers, 1982).

The operating temperature range is a function of the gauge alloy, backing material and adhesive. For commercially available strain gauges the temperature ranges mostly fit within the experimental temperature range for bone (-20 to $60°C$), although other ranges are available for specific high and low temperature applications.

For application to wet bone, strain gauges can be waterproofed by encapsulation and if a suitable adhesive is used the instrumented specimen can be immersed in Ringer's solution, facilitating the maintenance and manipulation of temperature throughout the experiment.

Pre-encapsulated gauges (e.g. Techni Measure, WFRA–1) are found to be convenient and offer many advantages including the elimination of gauge handling, soldering and insulation, the wiring of the harness complete with gauges providing a waterproof system and ease in bonding the strain gauge onto the bone surface.

There are disadvantages with pre-encapsulated gauges, for example, precise gauge alignment is more difficult, and they are more expensive. One material that has been used for the encapsulation is a semi-flexible polysulphide epoxy, with an upper temperature limit of 80°C. It is important that the encapsulation only covers the electrical wires and not the back of the gauge; the gauge backing needs to be in direct contact with the specimen so that the strain is transmitted from the test material via the adhesive to the gauge grid.

Resistance strain gauge theory assumes that the strain appearing in the gauge grid is identical to that occurring on the surface to which the gauge is bonded. It is very important to recognize the significant influence the adhesive has on the strain gauge properties such as gauge factor, creep performance, linearity, hysteresis and temperature response. Therefore proper adhesive selection and application are very important steps in the installation procedure. The ideal strain gauge adhesive should have minimum curing time, require no mixing, give only a thin layer, require low clamping pressure, have a wide temperature range, be insoluble in physiological saline and show linearity with minimal creep and hysteresis and high elongation capability. Cyanoacrylate is found to be most suitable as it is very fast curing and simple to use, possessing many of the characteristics mentioned above.

Application of strain gauges to bone may be summarized as follows: the specimen is defrosted at room temperature in Ringer's solution, removed from the solution and tissue dried so that only the surface moisture is removed. A drop of cyanoacrylate is applied to the marked surface and spread evenly into a thin film, and the back surface of the encapsulated strain gauge is attached onto the testing surface. Application of thumb pressure for 30s is sufficient for a strong bond, after which the instrumented specimen can be reimmersed in Ringer's solution. In order to reduce further dehydration of the specimen it is advisable to mark the location of the gauges before freezing. Series of tests have shown that this bond is not affected within the temperature range of −5°C to 55°C (Dabestani, 1989). Morden (1982) has shown that cyanoacrylate has a creep-free performance, and an elongation capability in the region of 15% strain (150 000 microstrain), which enables dynamic testing of bone within the physiological stress levels and strain rates, without any effects from the adhesive. The previous suggestions of Wright and Hayes (1979) such as scraping and degreasing of the bone surface are not necessary requirements for the installation of the strain gauges, and may be avoided. Employment of strain gauges can provide an efficient and accurate technique for *in vitro* strain measurement, taking certain points into account. Van Buskirk *et al*. (1981) advise against the measurement of anisotropy using separate specimens as it is impossible to fabricate multiple bone specimens with identical microstructure and ultrastructure. An alternative method is to use rosette strain gauges with multichannel strain measuring so that the readings from the three gauges of each rosette are recorded simultaneously (Dabestani and Bonfield, 1988). Two rosette gauges should be attached at either side of the specimen within the gauge length to eliminate bending effects and provide the comparison of the anisotropic strain data.

The choice of specimen thickness is restricted by the type of bone; for example, the maximum thickness of cortical bone specimens from human femora is approximately 2 mm. For thin specimens it is necessary to identify whether reinforcement effects are interfering with the results by independent calibration as has been discussed by Little in Chapter 3.

The attachment of strain gauges to whole bones is principally the same as for the specimens of bone. In this case the number and distribution of the gauges are dictated by the nature of the experiment, but the fundamental point is the alignment of the rosette gauges with the long axis which is done by eye, or using a suitable jig. As has been described by Bundy (1978) the mechanical properties of bone vary along the bone shaft as well as in the periphery. Thus the number and distribution of the gauges should provide an accurate analysis of the inhomogeneity and anisotropy. For example, on the human femur, five rows of rosette gauges applied to the medial, lateral and anterior aspects have been found to be adequate. Finlay *et al*. (1982) recommend that depending on the size of the bone between 22 and 25 rosette strain gauges can be arranged in five rows. However, Carter *et al*. (1981) have pointed out that for an accurate strain measurement the space between the rosette gauges around the bone circumference is very important, as greater gauge spacing results in larger strain differences making the analysis less sensitive to experimental errors but the reinforcing effect of the gauges needs to be considered. The data acquisition and instrumentation of such a set up is complex.

4.4. INSTRUMENTATION

The strain gauge itself is only a passive resistor, which requires activation. The strain gauge instrumentation consists of a bridge circuit which measures the changes in resistance caused by mechanical strain by producing an out-of-balance voltage which is then amplified and processed. The processing may be analogue, or in computer based systems, digital. For measurements of static strains commercially available strain indicators are suitable. Dynamic measurements from a few channels require the amplification of the analogue signals and simultaneous recording. For large test programmes elaborate computer based purpose built systems are available.

The initial step in strain gauge measurement is to balance the bridge, to compensate for resistance tolerances of the gauges and to account for environmental effects such as temperature. The signal from the strain gauge has to go through amplification before processing, manipulation and storage can be done. While with static measurements it is possible to use an amplifier together with a switch to incorporate a number of gauges in dynamic tests, correlation between different measurement points requires separate amplification for each channel (Scott and Owens, 1982).

The output signal is directly proportional to the strain change at the gauge position, but needs further processing to produce the strain reading. Analogue processing in strain gauge testing is generally the manipulation and testing of the output voltage. For digital processing, the analogue signals are passed through an analogue-to-digital converter into the computer. In dynamic testing, a high speed analogue-to-digital converter is necessary.

Real-time processing is limited by sampling speed and data storage but can be carried out whether analogue or digital data storage is used. In the latter case, the analogue processing is carried out before the analogue-to-digital conversion, and as analogue processing is generally faster than digital, the total processing time can be decreased and the maximum sampling rate increased.

In dynamic testing, large quantities of data can be recorded with analogue processing and stored in analogue form convenient for immediate visual analysis. Typical examples of analogue data storage systems are UV recorder, chart recorder, oscilloscope output, tape recorder, and numerical printout for low frequency (< 1 Hz) dynamic test (Scott and Owens, 1982). Lanyon *et al.* (1975) employed analogue signal processing extensively for *in vivo* strain measurements of bone.

The choice of system between analogue and digital is dependent on many factors. In dynamic testing sampling rate plays a vital part in establishing an accurate measure of strain, in particular with regard to the turning points, that is the peaks and troughs, of the cycle. In order to obtain adequate data and the turning points of each element of the rosette strain gauge, a minimum sampling rate of 10 points per cycle is recommended for all channels.

In summary, digital signal processing allows full exploitation of the computer's capability and numerical algorithms and for testing frequencies applied to bone between 1 and 5 Hz a more convenient technique for the quantitative assessment of the dynamic properties than the analogue signal processing.

4.5 DATA ANALYSIS

Analysis of rosette gauge data from isotropic materials is relatively straightforward as the orientation of the principal stresses is identical to those of the principal strains and the magnitude of the principal strains are calculated directly from gauge outputs. Stress analysis from anisotropic materials is more complex since the orientation of the principal strains is not the same as those of the principal stresses, and these relationships are dependent on the principal material axis.

It has been shown by Reilly and Burstein (1975) and Van Buskirk *et al.* (1981) that bone is at least transversely isotropic, that is it exhibits one set of elastic properties in one direction and a second set in the two directions perpendicular to that direction, and a minimum of five materials constants are required to define its elastic properties. A more comprehensive analysis of anisotropy can be considered by assuming orthotropy, that is three separate elastic moduli in the three material

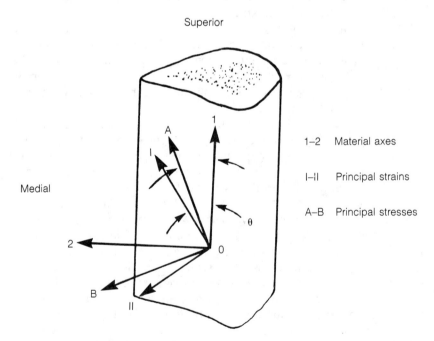

Figure 4.1 Reference axes for anistropic analysis (reprinted with permission from Carter (1978), *J. Biomech.*, **11**, 199–202, Pergamon Press).

directions, and nine distinct elastic constants are required to define the state of anisotropy in bone (Turner and Cowin, 1988). The assumption of transverse isotropy and the analysis following thereafter is by no means exhaustive.

Figure 4.1 shows the system of axes considered for the analysis of Carter (1978), from the rosette data at point 0:

- The principal material directions are 1 and 2.
- The directions of the principal strains are I and II.
- The directions of the principal stresses are A and B.
- Angle θ is between the principal strain axes and the material axes.
- Angle ϕ is between the principal stress axes and the material axes.

For a transversely isotropic analysis the strains in the principal material directions ϵ_1, ϵ_2 and ϵ_{12} are calculated using (Carter, 1978):

$$
\begin{vmatrix} \epsilon_1 \\ \epsilon_2 \\ \epsilon_{12} \end{vmatrix} = \begin{vmatrix} \cos^2\theta & \sin^2\theta & -2\sin\theta\,\cos\theta \\ \sin^2\theta & \cos^2\theta & 2\sin\theta\,\cos\theta \\ \sin\theta\,\cos\theta & -\sin\theta\,\cos\theta & \cos^2\theta - \sin^2\theta \end{vmatrix} \begin{vmatrix} \epsilon_I \\ \epsilon_{II} \\ 0 \end{vmatrix} \quad (4.1)
$$

The stresses in the principal material directions σ_1, σ_2 and σ_{12}:

$$
\begin{vmatrix} \sigma_1 \\ \sigma_2 \\ \sigma_{12} \end{vmatrix} = \begin{vmatrix} E_1 & \dfrac{-E_2}{v_{21}} & 0 \\ \dfrac{E_1}{v_{12}} & E_2 & 0 \\ 0 & 0 & 2G_{12} \end{vmatrix} \begin{vmatrix} \epsilon_1 \\ \epsilon_2 \\ \epsilon_{12} \end{vmatrix} \quad (4.2)
$$

where E_i is the elastic modulus in the ith direction, G_{ij} is the shear modulus in i-j plane, v_{ij} is Poisson's ratio in the j direction.

As has been described by Carter (1978) the magnitudes and directions of the principal stresses are found by

$$
\sigma_A, \sigma_B = \frac{\sigma_1 + \sigma_2}{2} \pm \sqrt{\left[\left(\frac{\sigma_1 - \sigma_2}{2} \right)^2 + \sigma_{12}^2 \right]} \quad (4.3)
$$

and

$$\phi = \frac{1}{2} \tan^{-1} \frac{2\sigma_{12}}{\sigma_1 - \sigma_2} \qquad (4.4)$$

It was further commented that the magnitudes and directions of principal stresses using anisotropic analysis differed significantly from those calculated using isotropic analysis. He thus recommended that strains and stresses estimated from rosettes bonded to bone should be reported in the principal material directions, since it is easier to integrate this information with gait and functional anatomy, and failure theories of composite materials including bone are based on stresses and strains in the principal material directions.

4.6 APPLICATION OF STRAIN GAUGES

Evans (1959) in early studies characterized compact bone as a truly elastic material with a linear stress–strain relationship to failure. Later contributions identified a yield behaviour while its exact position was in dispute; using extensometers Dempster and Liddicoat (1952) defined the yield point at approximately 50% of the final fracture stress. Frankel and Burstein (1965, 1970) and Burstein and Frankel (1968) demonstrated the existence of varying amounts of non-elastic strain at approximately 90% of the ultimate fracture stress.

Bonfield and Li (1966) using electrical resistance strain gauges and a microstrain sensitive measuring technique were able to detect small changes in strain well below the reported limits, whereby a microscopic yield stress (MYS) was defined at an average value of 0.5% of the ultimate tensile stress which provided 2×10^{-6} units of non-elastic strain (Bonfield and O'Connor, 1978). They further demonstrated that the deformation behaviour was composed of limited elastic deformation with a microscopic yield stress of 12 ± 8 MPa followed by a departure from linearity with a transition from a straight line load unload cycle to the formation of hysteresis loops. The non-elastic strain associated with the MYS was recoverable with time and was attributed entirely to anelastic deformation.

Wright and Yettram (1977) used electrical resistance strain gauges in order to study the effect of a standard femoral component on the distribution and magnitude of the longitudinal (axial) and circumferential (hoop) stresses induced in the supporting femoral bone. Strain gauges were attached to both medial and lateral bone surfaces and the medial and lateral aspects of the femoral component. The strain gauge measurements were recorded on paper tape. They concluded that in the calcar region the magnitude of the stress appeared to be dependent upon the contact of the metal collar with the medial cortex, and with no contact the stresses in the calcar were very small. They therefore proposed a collar on all femoral components so as to ensure adequate load carrying by the calcar.

Schartzer *et al.* (1978) used strain gauges to quantify the stress protection produced by internal fixation of fractures. The bones were strain gauged *in vitro* and loaded to determine the ratio of applied load and strain. The bone was then resected and repaired either by internal fixation plates for transverse osteotomies either with or without compression or for oblique osteotomies by 'lag' screws. The loading was repeated and the relationship between load and strain was again determined. They found that the lag screws provided no stress protection but that the internal fixation plates reduced the strain measured by the strain gauges. The amount of stress protection was not dependent on the amount of compression but was affected by the stiffness of the plate.

Currey and Horsman (1981) applied four rosette strain gauges, two 25 mm and a further two 70 mm above the styloid process of female radii whose bone mineral content had been measured using an absorptiometric system. They found inverse relationships between the strain at 600 N load and the bone mineral content, with higher strains in the area just below the styloid process for a given mineral content. The average ratio of the strains was 1.7:1 with the higher strains being in the areas with more cancellous bone.

Dabestani (1989) using encapsulated rosette strain gauges subsequently developed an experimental microstrain measuring technique in order to investigate the dynamic and anisotropic properties of human compact bone, while maintaining the physiological conditions such as moisture state, temperature, stress levels and strain rate. It was demonstrated that modelling of compact bone based on the elastic performance is inadequate, since the deformation in bone is dominantly anelastic and affected by the anisotropic properties. It was also shown that the dynamic response of compact bone is viscoelastic which is a factor that needs to be involved in modelling a successful replacement material.

4.7 CONCLUSIONS

Strain gauges offer versatility and can be used in a wide variety of studies. They also permit the maintenance of physiological conditions such as temperature and moisture content while including test requirements like stress levels and strain rates. Other advantages include anisotropic analysis, direct and continuous measurement of strain and the choice of signal processing makes them a convenient method for quantitative assessment of dynamic properties of bone.

REFERENCES

Abenschein, W.G. and Hyatt, G.W. (1970) Ultrasonic and selected physical properties of bone. *Clin. Orthop.*, **69**, 294–301.

Baggott, D.G. and Lanyon, L.E. (1977) An independent post mortem calibration of electrical resistance strain gauges bonded to bone surfaces *in vivo*. *J. Biomech.*, **10**, 615–22.

Bonfield, W. and Clark, A.E. (1973) Elastic deformation of compact bone. *J. Mater. Sci.*, **8**, 1590–4.

Bonfield, W., Datta, P.K., Edwards, B.L. and Plane, D.C. (1973) A capacitance gauge for microstrain measurement. *J. Mater. Sci.*, **8**, 1832–4.

Bonfield, W. and Li, C.H. (1966) Deformation and fracture of bone. *J. Appl. Phys.*, **3**, 869–74.

Bonfield, W. and O'Connor, P.A. (1978) Anelastic deformation and the friction stress of bone. *J. Mater. Sci.*, **13**, 202–7.

Bundy, K.J. (1978) Experimental studies of the non-uniformity and anisotropy of human compact bone, PhD thesis, Stanford University.

Burstein, A.H. and Frankel, V.H. (1968) The viscoelastic properties of some biological materials. *Ann. N.Y. Acad. Sci.*, **146**, 158–65.

Carter, D.R. (1978) Anisotropic analysis of strain rosette information from cortical bone. *J. Biomech.*, **11**, 199–202.

Carter, D.R., Caler, W.E. and Harris, W.H. (1981) Resultant loads and elastic modulus calibration of long bone cross sections. *J. Biomech.*, **14**, 739–45.

Chalmers, G.F. (1982) Materials, construction, performance and characteristics, in *Strain Gauge Technology* (eds A.L. Window and G.S. Holister), Applied Science Publishers, Barking, pp. 20–5.

Currey, J.D. (1988) The effect of drying and re-wetting on some mechanical properties of cortical bone. *J. Biomech.*, **21**, 439–41.

Currey, J.D. and Horsman, A. (1981) Strength of the distal radius, in *Mechanical Factors and the Skeleton* (ed. I.A.F. Stokes), John Libbey, London, pp. 91–7.

Dabestani, M. (1989) The deformation behaviour of human compact bone, PhD thesis, University of London.

Dabestani, M. and Bonfield, W. (1988) Elastic and anelastic microstrain measurement in human and cortical bone, in *Implant Materials in Biofunction* (eds C. de Putter, G.L. de Lange, K. de Groot and A.J.C. Lee), Elsevier Science Publishers, Oxford, pp. 435–40.

Dempster, W.T. and Liddicoat, R.T. (1952) Compact bone as a non-isotropic material. *Am. J. Anat.*, **91**, 331–62.

Evans, F.G. (1959) *The Mechanical Properties of Bone*, 1st edn, C.C. Thomas, Springfield, IL., p. 11.

Evans, F.G. (1973) *The Mechanical Properties of Bone*, 2nd edn, C.C. Thomas, Springfield, IL., p. 2.

Finlay, J.B., Bourne, R.B. and McLean, J. (1982) A technique for the *in vitro* measurement of principal strains in human tibia. *J. Biomech.*, **15**, 723–39.

Frankel, V.H. and Burstein, A.H. (1965) In *Biomechanics and Related Bioengineering Topics* (ed. R.M. Kennedi), Pergamon Press, Oxford, p. 381.

Frankel, V.H. and Burstein, A.H. (1970) *Orthopaedic Biomechanics*, Lea and Fabiger, Philadelphia, PA.

Greenberg, S.W., Gonzalez, G., Gurdjian, E.S. and Thomas, L.M. (1968) Changes in physical properties of bone between the *in vivo*, freshly dead and embalmed conditions. *Proceedings of 12th Stapp Car Crash Conference*, Society of Automotive Engineers, New York, pp. 271–9.

Guardian, E.S. and Lissner, H.R. (1945) Deformation of the skull in head injury. A study with the stress coat technique. *Surg., Gyn. Obst.*, **81**, 679–87.

Lanyon, L.E., Hampson, W.G.J., Goodship, A.E. and Shah, J.S. (1975) Bone deformation recorded *in vivo* from strain gauges attached to the human tibial shaft. *Acta Orthop. Scand.*, **46**, 256–68.

Lissner, H.R. and Roberts, V.L. (1966) Evaluation of skeletal implants of human cadavers, in *Studies on the Anatomy and Function of Bone and Joints* (ed. F.G. Evans), Springer-Verlag, Heidelberg, pp. 113–20.

Manley, M.T., Ovryn, B. and Stern, L.S. (1987) Evaluation of double-exposure holographic interferometry for biomechanical measurements *in vitro*. *J. Orthop. Res.*, **5**, 144–9.

Milch, H. (1940) Photoelastic studies of bone forms. *J. Bone Jt Surg.*, **22–A**, 621–6.

Morden, G.C. (1982) Adhesives and installation techniques, in *Strain Gauge Technology* (eds A.L. Window and G.S. Holister), Applied Science Publishers, Barking, pp. 43–54.

Pelker, R.R., Friedlaender, G.E., Markham, T.C., Panjabi, M.M. and Moen, C.J. (1984) Effects of freezing and freeze-drying on the biomechanical properties of rat bone. *J. Orthop. Res.*, **1**, 405–11.

Reilly, D.T. and Burstein, A.H. (1975) The elastic and ultimate properties of compact bone tissue. *J. Biomech.*, **8**, 393–405.

Schartzer, J., Sumner-Smith, G., Clark, R. and McBroom, R. (1978) Strain gauge analysis of bone response to internal fixation. *Clin. Orthop.*, **132**, 244–51.

Scott, K. and Owens, A. (1982) Instrumentation, in *Strain Gauge Technology* (eds A.L. Window and G.S. Holister), Applied Science Publishers, Barking, pp. 139–41, 169–79.

Seldin, E.D. and Hirsch, C. (1966) Factors affecting the determination of the physical properties of femoral cortical bone. *Acta Orthop. Scand.*, **37**, 29–48.

Stevens, J. and Ray, R.D. (1962) An experimental comparison of living and dead bone in rats 1, physical properties. *J. Bone Jt Surg.*, **44–B**, 412–3.

Turner, C.H. and Cowin, S.C. (1988) Errors induced by off-axis measurement of the elastic properties of bone. *J. Biomech. Engng.*, **110**, 213–19.

Van Buskirk, W.C., Cowin, S.C. and Ward, R.N. (1981) Ultrasonic measurement of orthopaedic elastic constants of bovine femoral bone. *J. Biomech. Engng*, **103**, 67–71.

Wertheim, M.G. (1847) Memoires sur l'elasticite et la cohesion des principaux tissues de corps humain. *Annales de Chimie et de Physique (Paris)*, **21**, 385–414.

Wright, T.M. and Hayes, W.C. (1979) Strain gauge applications on compact bone. *J. Biomech.*, **12**, 471–5.

Wright, K.W.J. and Yettram, A.L. (1977) The transmission of force by the femoral component of a total hip replacement. Conference on Interdisciplinary Trends in Surgery, European Congress of International College of Surgeons, Milan, Italy.

5

The measurement of bone strain *in vivo*

A.E. Goodship

5.1 INTRODUCTION

Quantification of the stresses induced in structures by normal and abnormal loading is a standard requirement in many branches of engineering. By utilizing techniques of theoretical modelling or by direct measurement, the appropriate shape, size and materials can be determined for structures in relation to their functional requirements.

In the relatively young discipline of bio-engineering, one of the more important load bearing structures in the body is the skeleton. It is important to understand the dynamic biomechanics of this structure in order to design appropriate methods for repair of fractured bones and prostheses for replacement of skeletal components. As a load bearing structure the skeleton is somewhat unique in that it can respond to changes in mechanical demand. In a biological system the cost of support and movement in terms of energy expenditure is highly significant. The mass and distribution of bone must be closely related to the magnitude and direction of applied loads, allowing for occasional overload without a high risk of failure but minimizing mass to reduce energy requirements.

This interesting dynamic relationship between form and function is common in living structures and exemplified in the skeleton. About a century ago both engineers and biologists noted the order in bone form, in particular the arrangement of internal bony struts, trabeculae, in the proximal femur, Figure 5.1. These trabeculae form arcades that lie in a position similar to the stress trajectories calculated for a structure of like shape and loaded in the same manner, the Fairbairn crane, Figure 5.2. This and other observations on change in bone morphology resulting from changes in functional use led Julius Wolff (1892) to formulate his classic law of bone remodelling. This law incorporated two concepts, first that the architecture of a bone is adjusted to best

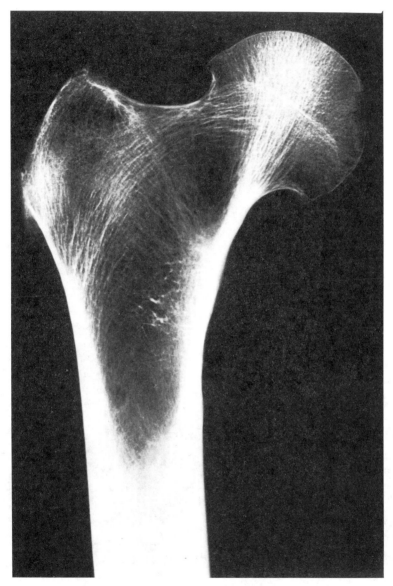

Figure 5.1 A radiograph of the proximal femur illustrating the arrangements of trabecular arcades.

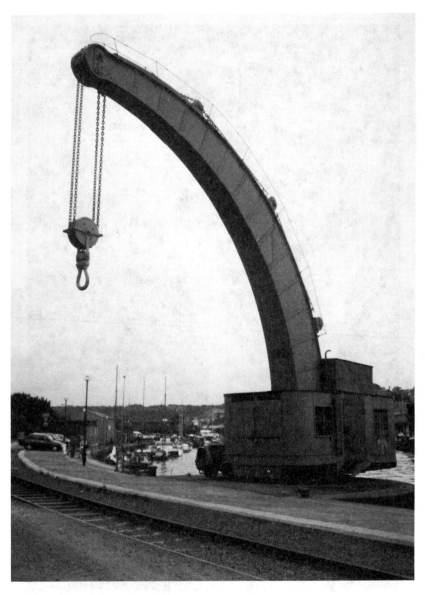

Figure 5.2 A Fairbairn crane as an example of a man-made structure loaded in a similar manner to that in the femur.

withstand the prevailing loads and secondly, that the mass of the skeletal element will be appropriate for the magnitude of the currently applied loads. The hypothesis put forward by Wolff was based on observations of changes in bone form and assumptions regarding the changes in the prevailing mechanical environment. An understanding of stress related remodelling is vital, not only to determine the functional stresses of the skeleton but also to determine, in a predictable manner, the influence of an orthopaedic implant on the normal mechanical environment and the consequent biological response to the presence of such an implant.

Bone as both an organ and a tissue is not an inert material, it is highly dynamic and remodels in response to various stimuli throughout life. One of the most important and potent of these stimuli is, in broad terms, the prevailing mechanical environment. Changes in the shape and size of the bone are brought about by an integrated response of the extracellular matrix and the three cell types involved in the removal, formation and maintenance of bone tissue to the perceived mechanical demands (Skerry *et al.*, 1988, 1990).

To verify Wolff's hypotheses it is necessary to quantify both the prevailing mechanical environment and the resultant biological response. Analysis of stress or strain distribution in bone has been attempted using computer modelling, photoelastic studies on plastic models of bone or by photoelastic coating of cadaveric specimens, the use of stress coat lacquers and attachment of strain gauges to postmortem samples. In all these techniques the strain magnitude and distribution will depend upon the size and direction of the applied loads. A realistic estimation of these values in relation to physiological loading is extremely difficult and has been discussed in Chapter 2 of this book. The complex arrangement of muscles, tendons and ligaments combined with the diversity of applied loads during different normal activities precludes an accurate determination of this variable.

In order to address the question of how mechanical environment influences the structure and shape of adult bone it is essential to quantify some aspect of the mechanical environment of living bone during normal activities. This was made possible with the advent of the technique of attaching strain gauges to living bone during physiological activities in the late 1960s (Lanyon and Smith, 1969). The direct measurement of strain or deformation resulting from the complex interaction of muscular and gravitational forces necessitated a gauge configuration that would provide data that could be used to calculate both the magnitude and orientation of the principal strains. Consequently it became apparent that as the orientation of principal strains could not be accurately predicted, and indeed may change in relation to different types of activity, it was imperative that a rosette strain gauge configuration be used. This would itself have limitations in that the data would only provide information relating to a small area at a single location on the bone. Nevertheless the development of this technique for *in vivo* recording was a vital step forward and provided the potential to relate form to function in a quantitative manner. By utilizing a number of rosettes around the circumference of a bone together with measurement of the second moment of area it is possible to calculate the loading characteristics at that plane during physiological activity. The use of strain measurements *in vivo* may be applied not only to bone itself but also to orthopaedic implants used in the repair and replacement of skeletal elements. Thus this technique can be used to advance understanding of strain related remodelling in normal bone and also the response of repair and remodelling in relation to the presence of implants. These data can then be utilized in the improvement of the functional compatibility of orthopaedic devices and possibly provide the basis for credible computer modelling to screen new designs of prostheses.

5.2 THE TECHNIQUE OF *IN VIVO* BONE STRAIN MEASUREMENT

The successful use of conventional strain gauges to determine the functional deformations occurring in living bone depends upon two factors: first, the modification of the gauge to withstand the hostile environment of the body and, second, the reliable bonding of the gauge to the bone such that it deforms as if part of the skeletal structure for a reasonable period of time. Implantation and attachment of such gauges to bone *in vivo* was first achieved independently by Lanyon and Smith (1969, 1970), Lanyon (1972) and Cochran (1972) in the early 1970s. This technique has evolved to be used extensively in biomechanical investigations of the skeleton in relation to remodelling, repair and development of replacement prostheses.

The technique utilizes standard 45° foil rosette gauges as used in more conventional engineering applications, Figure 5.3. For biological implantation the gauges have to be modified and protected from the conducting salt solutions forming the body fluids. The gauges as received have first to be attached to fine PTFE lead wires which, to reduce the risk of fatigue failure, are then joined to more substantial PTFE insulated wires within a small epoxy resin junction block a short distance from the gauge. The junction block itself is attached to the bone cortex by means of a cortical bone screw. The larger diameter lead wires are taken subcutaneously to emerge at a convenient point through a separate incision. After exposing the site to be instrumented the periosteum has to be removed over the area to which the gauge

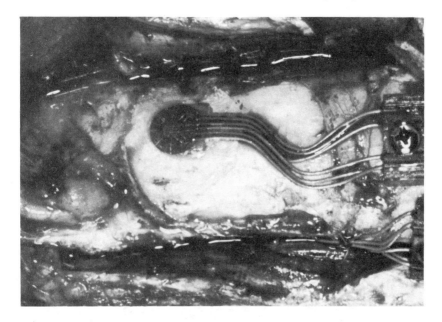

Figure 5.3 A rosette strain gauge unit bonded to living bone after removal of the periosteum.

will be applied. The surface of the bone must be clean and complete haemostasis achieved, the surface of the bone is then degreased using a small amount of diethyl ether. Once the site has been adequately prepared a few drops of cyanoacrylate adhesive are applied to the back of the gauge unit and the gauges firmly pressed onto the bone surface using a polyethylene finger stool. A satisfactory bond is usually achieved after a period of about 1 min. The surgical wound is closed using standard suturing procedures.

Recordings can be taken over a period of up to 12 weeks, although the working life of the unit may be considerably less. Each element of the rosette forms part of a standard Wheatstone bridge circuit and is used in a quarter bridge configuration. During physiological activities the rates of change in strain magnitude vary during the loading cycle, so the point of least deformation may be difficult to define. In locomotion the bones of the limbs are deformed at the greatest rate during the transition from swing to stance phase of gait. Minimal rate of change in strain occurs during the swing phase, Figure 5.4, some researchers therefore define the strain levels recorded during the swing phase as the physiological zero strain level. The alternative method of defining a zero point is to consider the value measured when the subject is anaesthetized. Although muscles are relaxed under anaesthesia in terms of the functional mechanical environment and its influence on

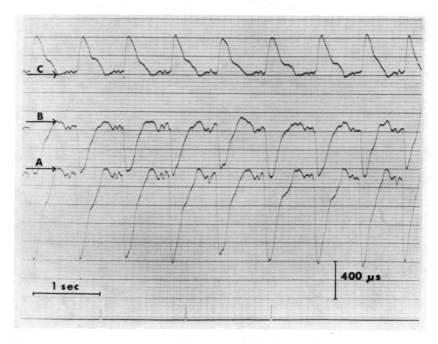

Figure 5.4 Typical recordings from each element of a rosette strain gauge during normal locomotion. The arrows indicate physiological zero levels during the period of low rate of change in swing phase of gait.

bone remodelling, such a state is non-physiological and thus may not be the most appropriate zero reference. The problem is greater in bones that are not subjected to an easily defined loading cycle.

Using calibration resistors enables the technique to be used to determine absolute strain values provided the gauge to bone bond is adequate and reliable. It has been shown that gauges implanted for 12 weeks *in vivo* still provided data that correlated to within 1% of values obtained using mirror extensometers in post-mortem calibration experiments. Thus the technique is reliable, reproducible and accurate.

5.3 *IN VIVO* STRAIN MEASUREMENTS AND THE FUNCTIONAL ENVIRONMENT OF THE SKELETON

The use of *in vivo* strain measurement to establish functional environments has been used as a technique to investigate the validity of Wolff's hypotheses. In terms of the relationship between the architecture of skeletal elements and the direction of applied loads it would be difficult to instrument the proximal femur of the human. In quadrupeds such as the sheep the os calcis or heel bone acts as a simple cantilever, being loaded by the Achilles tendon complex. Radiographs of this bone show an internal architecture comprising two main trabecular arcades, one in the dorsal region of the bone and the other in the plantar position. The trabecular arcades intersect in an orthogonal manner. Lanyon (1974) showed that the orientation of principal strains measured at various sites on the lateral surface of this bone correlated with the direction of the trabecular arcades within the bone. Minimal principal strains were aligned with the dorsal arcade of trabeculae and maximal principal strains with the plantar arcade. This experiment provides some circumstantial evidence for the trajectorial concept initiated by Wolff. Confirmation of a causal relationshp would require some perturbation of the system to demonstrate a correlation between changed loading direction and subsequent trabecular remodelling.

Strain gauges have also been used *in vivo* to determine the functional loading patterns for specific bones. The accuracy of such investigations is related to the number of gauges applied at the level of interest together with the accuracy of measurement of the geometry and material properties of the bone at that site. Information on functional loading may be of value not only in understanding the relationships between form and function in the skeleton but also in defining the optimal position for implants in the repair and replacement of specific skeletal elements. The functional loading of the radius in quadrupeds has been shown to include compression and bending, whereas in the tibia of many animals including man, there is a significant torsional component (Lanyon *et al.*, 1975; Rubin and Lanyon, 1982). Such data can only be obtained from direct *in vivo* strain measurement due to the complex interactions of muscles. The technique provides the opportunity to verify or correct some of the mathematical models relating to the biomechanics of the skeleton.

5.4 THE INFLUENCE OF FUNCTIONAL STRAINS ON ADAPTIVE REMODELLING OF THE SKELETON

Strain levels have been measured in a number of species including man at various sites on different bones and it has been noted that the level of the principal strains during peak physiological activity were in the same order of magnitude (Rubin and Lanyon, 1984). The similarity of strain levels appears to be independent of anatomical conformation or the histological structure of the bone, Table 5.1. This apparent universal level of customary strain presents the possible hypothesis that bone mass is regulated to provide such strain levels in response to the loading demands at a given time. Any change in loading regime will alter the prevailing strain environment and provide a stimulus for remodelling and reorganization of bone tissue. This adaptive response may occur generally throughout the skeleton or be localized to one limb, bone or region within a bone. For example in professional tennis players it has been shown that the bone mass of the humerus in the serving arm may be 30% greater than that of the non-serving arm. Conversely in astronauts undertaking prolonged space flights there is a general loss of skeletal mass; approximately 10% bone loss may occur during a 100 day period in space. It is interesting, however, that this loss was not uniform throughout the skeleton but greater in bones subjected to less exercise, such as the lower limbs, than those in the upper limbs which were subjected to diverse loading whilst performing various tasks. In these situations it is not possible to quantify the change in mechanical environment. Experimental evidence obtained using strain gauges to quantify strain supports these responses to changed customary strain levels (Jones *et al.*, 1977; Goodship *et al.*, 1979; Stupakov *et al.*, 1984; Lanyon, 1987; Rubin and Lanyon, 1987). Removal of the ulna, one of a pair of bones in the forelimb, of a pig resulted in a 50% reduction of total cross-sectional area and an approximate doubling on strain levels on the remaining radius. Following a 3-month period of remodelling the radius showed both hypertrophy and a change in shape, at this time the cross-sectional area of bone had been restored to that of both radius and ulna in the contralateral limb together with a reduction in functional strain magnitudes to equate with those on the contralateral radius. The sensitivity of the response to change in strain environment was shown in similar experiments inducing increases in strain of only 5%.

Table 5.1 Peak functional strains measured from bone bonded strain gauges in a range of animals, during their customary activity which elicited the highest recorded strains (Rubin, 1982)

Bone	Activity	Peak strain recorded (microstrain)
Horse radius	Trotting	−2800
Horse tibia	Galloping	−3200
Horse metacarpal	Accelerating	−3000
Dog radius	Trotting	−2400
Dog tibia	Galloping	−2100
Goose humerus	Flying	−2800
Cockerel ulna	Flapping	−2100
Sheep femur	Trotting	−2200
Sheep humerus	Trotting	−2200
Sheep radius	Galloping	−2300
Sheep tibia	Trotting	−2100
Pig radius	Trotting	−2400
Fish hypural	Swimming	−3000
Macaca mandible	Biting	−2200

The ability to control the functional environment of a bone yet retain the influences of other aspects of functional environment such as blood flow and systemic hormones was achieved with the development of the isolated avian ulna model (Lanyon and Rubin, 1984). In this preparation a long bone could be isolated from normal functional loading within the wing of a bird, the remaining radius providing structural support for the wing. Furthermore, using orthopaedic pins transfixing the ends of the isolated bone shaft and emerging through the skin, similar to the pins used to apply traction in the treatment of fractures, the bone could be protected from incidental loading with an external fixator or subjected to controlled loading by attachment of an hydraulic actuator to the pins. Using this preparation, Lanyon and Rubin (1984) were able to demonstrate that only relatively few cycles of an osteogenic strain regime were required on a daily basis to evoke a remodelling response. Isolation of the bone resulted in the expected strain protection and consequent reduction in mass; however, only 36 strain cycles per day were necessary to cause hypertrophy of the bone and an increase above the 36 cycles did not produce a greater response. Again using this preparation Lanyon and Rubin (1984) confirmed earlier work of Hĕrt *et al.* (1971) to show that bone responds to intermittent or cyclical loads rather than static loading. The mechanisms involved in the transduction of the strain environment to cellular activity and remodelling are far from clear. Skerry *et al.* (1990) showed that changes can be observed in the orientation of proteoglycans in the extracellular matrix of bone, maximum effect was achieved after as few as 50 loading cycles and persisted for 48 h after cessation of loading. Since proteoglycans are present near the osteocyte lacunae and indeed may link with the cytoskeleton of the cell Skerry postulated that the changes in the matrix induced by loading may form a 'strain memory' and thus provide a template for structural remodelling should the strain environment change in a similar manner on a consistent basis. This would support the concept that bone remodelling is an error driven response. Skerry also showed that the cellular response to change in strain environment is extremely rapid. Within a few minutes of the application of an episode of an osteogenic strain regime the cells within the bone matrix (osteocytes) showed an increase in metabolism. This increase in cell activity in response to loading was not associated with cell division, since these cells are trapped within a hard matrix and cannot divide. The author suggested that the increase in metabolism was related to the synthesis of messenger molecules that would act in cell to cell signalling, both between osteocytes and osteocytes within the bone and osteoblasts on the bone surfaces that are associated with the control of bone remodelling. The osteoblasts on bone surfaces showed increased activity within a few days of a single period of loading. These data demonstrate the acutely sensitive response of the skeleton to changes in mechanical circumstance. Obviously mechanical factors, although of prime importance, are not the only aspect of functional environment that will influence bone remodelling. Vascular and hormonal factors will also play a part in the regulation of skeletal mass and may interact to modulate the response of the skeleton to mechanical loading. The sudden change in hormonal environment following the menopause appears to suppress the ability of the skeleton to withstand and respond to functional loading. The condition of osteoporosis now presents a significant clinical problem in our ageing population. Loss of bone material in both cortical and trabecular sites can occur to such an extent that normal loading results in fracture of the femoral neck, distal radius and collapse of vertebral bodies. Treatment of this condition has related largely to hormone replacement therapy and dietary factors and only recently has the role of mechanical stimulation gained attention. There is now some evidence that the loss of bone mass in these patients can be reduced or even reversed by providing an exercise regime based on high intensity diverse loading. This again indicates the potency of change in strain distribution as an osteogenic stimulus and provides further evidence for an error driven mechanism for bone remodelling.

5.5 THE ROLE OF STRAIN IN FRACTURE REPAIR

Many of the cells involved in the process of repair following fracture of bone are derived from the same sources as those responsible for the initial ossification and subsequent remodelling of the intact skeleton. Therefore perhaps it is not surprising that the repair process is also influenced by the prevailing mechanical environment. Both the amount and distribution of bone formed during repair are influenced by the magnitudes and distributions of strain at the fracture site.

Two major patterns of repair occur in bone depending upon the degree of stability of the fragments. Fixation with very rigid devices will result in a high level of stability and little or no relative movement between fragments. In this situation healing is slow and under ideal conditions of perfect reduction involves osteonal remodelling across the fracture line. In clinical situations 100% bone contact may not be achieved throughout the fracture line and in areas where gaps exist the strain levels may be high and preclude bone formation. No periosteal callus is seen in this type of healing and a good anatomical reconstruction is achieved. The process is termed direct or primary bone repair and is usually associated with the use of a rigid internal fixation plate and interfragmentary compression. An additional complication in this type of healing is the development of an intracortical porosity and some endosteal resorption. The porosity was originally attributed to strain protection afforded by load sharing with the fracture plate, and indeed strain gauge studies confirm that the cortex beneath a fracture plate experiences a reduction in strain during functional loading (Baggot *et al.*, 1981; Woo *et al.*, 1984). However, the presence of a plate adjacent to the periosteum also compromises the vasculature in that region and studies using plates with modified undersurfaces (Burny *et al.*, 1978) or the use of external fixators to induce strain protection confirm that the early porosis can be a result of vascular effects, whereas it is likely that endosteal resorption is linked to reduced mechanical demand (Butler *et al.*, 1991). Indeed in engineering terms such responses would have some credibility, maximizing strength with reduced material in a tubular structure may be better achieved by creating a thin walled large diameter tube than inducing porosity in the wall of the tube.

The second type of fracture repair is termed indirect or secondary bone healing and is characterized by the production of external periosteal callus which forms rapidly and acts as a biological supporting splint, Figure 5.5. This type of repair occurs in situations where there is a greater degree of interfragmentary strain or micromovement. Within this second pattern of repair the extent and distribution of callus are determined largely by the mechanical environment imposed by the fixation device. This type of repair process results in rapid restoration of mechanical integrity but requires a longer period of time to remodel the callus and achieve the original anatomical form of the bone. Indirect fracture repair results following the use of casts, braces, intramedullary nailing and external skeletal fixation.

Recently external fixation has gained popularity as a method of fracture management, it can allow greater patient mobility than casts; the frame stiffness and rigidity can be varied without further surgical intervention and soft tissue injuries are accessible for treatment. However, the full potential to utilize external fixators to achieve the optimal environment for maximal healing has not yet been realized in the clinical field.

Following fracture the functional use of the limb is reduced and the bone is afforded additional support by one of the treatment regimes outlined above. These events reduce or remove the osteogenic mechanical stimulus at the very time when rapid new bone formation is required. It would appear logical therefore to attempt to provide both support for the fractured bone and an appropriate stimulus for bone formation at the same time. The rate and extent of callus formation is determined indirectly by the stiffness and rigidity of the frame; clinically frames appear to be applied with little consideration for these variables yet experimentally there is evidence that the pattern of healing can be significantly influenced by these frame variables. This

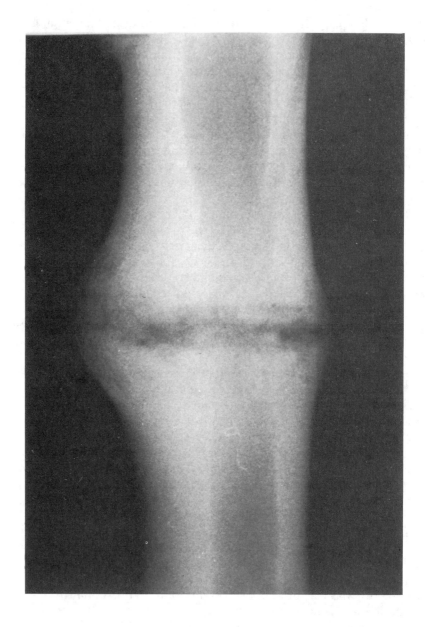

Figure 5.5 A radiograph to illustrate indirect bone healing, the stabilization of bone fragments following osteotomy is achieved by bridging callus on both endosteal and periosteal surfaces.

indicates a need to define the frame properties *in situ* and utilize the ability to change frame configuration to influence healing in a controlled manner. Measurement of frame deformation using strain gauges has been developed (Burny *et al.*, 1978; Evans *et al.*, 1988) both as a method of objective assessment of restoration of the mechanical integrity of the fractured bone, and also to allow removal or restructuring of the frame at a mechanically appropriate point.

One of the problems with external fixation relates to the pin-bone and pin-skin interfaces. Although a device with low stiffness and rigidity will permit greater interfragmentary movement and stimulate more bone formation, the flexion of the pins results in pin-tract infection and the potential for high stresses at the pin-bone interface which may lead to bone resorption and pin loosening (Pope and Evans, 1982). These problems can be overcome using frames with high stiffness and rigidity, however, these afford greater strain protection at the fracture site and consequently inhibit healing. Since remodelling in intact bone can be evoked by very short periods of daily loading the effect of applying a similar stimulus to healing fractures was used in an attempt to combine the beneficial effects of rigid frames with an adequate osteogenic stimulus. The influence of the applied micromovement on restoration of mechanical integrity was assessed using a measure of fracture stiffness index at intervals after fixation (Goodship and Kenwright, 1985). The stiffness index was obtained from simultaneous recordings from strain transducers attached to the fixator column and vertical ground reaction forces from a Kistler force plate. The concept of using strain gauges bonded to orthopaedic devices to evaluate the progression of healing in patients was pioneered by Burny *et al.* (1978), other workers have developed the technique to allow groups of patients to be evaluated and compared (Kenwright *et al.*, 1986).

Using an osteotomy model in sheep stabilized with a rigid external fixator, it has been shown that as few as 500 cycles of interfragmentary movement applied at 0.5 Hz each day can significantly affect the progression of healing compared with a rigid control (Kenwright and Goodship, 1989). Furthermore, within the short period of imposed micromovement variation of displacement magnitude, rate and initial maximum stress can themselves result in significant effects on healing. In these experiments it was found that interfragmenary micromovement applied with low levels of initial displacement, low stress and high rates of movement resulted in significant increases in the rate of healing. The experimental findings were extended to human patients in a controlled clinical trail at two centres and the experimental results were found to be valid in human patients with significant improvements in healing being achieved with applied mechanical stimulation (Kenwright and Goodship, 1989). The most important criterion for determining the end point of healing must be restoration of mechanical integrity and it is now possible using strain gauges to define the levels of fracture stiffness at which there is minimal risk of refracture when the fixator is removed.

5.6 *IN VIVO* STRAIN MEASUREMENT AND THE DESIGN OF PROSTHESES

The materials from which prostheses are constructed are tested for biocompatibility, however, such tests relate largely to potential toxic effects on biological tissues. Perhaps one of the most successful joint replacement prostheses is the total hip, yet even with modern technology for design and selection of materials this prosthesis has a limited life before adverse bone remodelling leads to loosening and the need for revision surgery. The increase in life expectancy and demand for high quality of life means that today joint replacements may be performed earlier and have to last longer than the initial replacements. Even in cases where there is excellent surgical technique and no infection the loosening rate increases with time. In many cases this loosening results from adverse bone remodelling. Bone is resorbed from the proximal region of the femur and the initial support for the prosthesis is lost, progressive interfacial micromovement occurs and the prosthesis loosens. Other complications such as cellular reaction in response to wear debris may exacerbate the rate of loosening. The insertion of a synthetic prosthesis into the medullary canal of the femur changes the load transfer and resultant strain distributions in the proximal femur. This change in strain environment will initiate a remodelling response resulting in a change in bone mass and distribution, thus the functional compatibility is far from satisfactory, the ability of an implant to integrate with bone in a functional manner must be as important as its safety from a toxicological viewpoint. However, little consideration has been paid to the relationship between prosthetic design and functional bone strains. The biological concept of functional compatibility in terms of strain environment can be tested in animal models, however, there is no animal in which the hip joint is identical to that of the human. Nor is it easy to calculate the magnitudes and distributions of the strains in the human femur during physiological activity. In experimental studies using implanted strain gauges it can be shown that both the magnitude and orientation of principal strains in the proximal femur are altered following insertion of both cemented and uncemented femoral components (Lanyon *et al.*, 1981). In the region of the calcar the minimum principal strain is reduced and hoop strains are increased, the resultant effect on bone remodelling is resorption of the calcar. If the limb is not loaded then there is generalized cortical thinning without specific calcar resorption, this suggests that the stimulus for remodelling is largely attributable to the change in strain distribution. These studies would suggest that design criteria for prostheses should include functional strain compatibility and possibly aim to create osteogenic strain patterns in areas where bone is required to provide long term support for prostheses. The behaviour of the implant can also be monitored by the application of strain gauges. The problems associated with percutaneous leads have to be overcome, modern electronic technology has made the possibility of implantable externally powered telemetry, as discussed in Chapter 6, a feasible option. The use of strain gauges in this way should yield unique data on the functional behaviour of the implant; since attachment of gauges to bone involves removal of periosteum long term implantation will inevitably compromise remodelling activity. This together with the small area covered by any one gauge represents some of the limitations of the technique of *in vivo* strain measurement.

5.7 CONCLUSIONS

Notwithstanding the limitations discussed in this chapter, the technique of *in vivo* strain measurement still represents a significant advance in direct quantification of the normal mechanical environment of the skeleton. It has contributed significantly to the understanding of Wolff's postulates in relation to the equilibrium between functional demands and the remodelling, repair and replacement of the bones of the skeleton. This technique should also provide data to enhance the credibility of computer modelling of biomechanics in relation to the skeleton, and in the long term, enable the development of mathematical analysis that will eliminate, or at least diminish, the need for *in vivo* measurements.

REFERENCES

Baggot, D.G., Goodship, A.E. and Lanyon, L.E. (1981) A quantitative assessment of compression plate fixation *in vivo* an experimental study using sheep radius. *J. Biomech.*, **14** (10), 701–11.

Burny, F., Bourgois, R., Donkerwolcke, M. and Moulart, F. (1978) Utilisation clinique de jauges de constrainte – situation actuelle et prosectures d'avenir. *Acta Orthop. Belg.*, **44**, 895–920.

Butler, S.P., O'Doherty, D. and Goodship, A. E. (1991) Stress protection of the sheep tibia using an Oxford Mk II external fixator. *Proc. Brit. Orthop. Res. Soc.*, *J. Bone Jt Surg.* (in press).

Cochran, G.V.B. (1972) Implantation of strain gauges *in vivo*. *J. Biomech.*, **5**, 119–23.

Evans, M., Kenwright, J. and Cunningham, J.L. (1988) Design and performance of a fracture monitoring transducer. *J. Biomed. Engng.*, **10**, 64.

Goodship, A.E. and Kenwright, J. (1985) The influence of induced micromovement upon healing of experimental tibial fractures. *J. Bone Jt Surg.*, **67B** (4), 650–5.

Goodship, A.E., Lanyon, L.E. and McFie, H. (1979) Functional adaptation of bone to increased stress. *J. Bone Jt. Surg.*, **61-A**, 539–46.

Hĕrt, J., Lishova, M. and Landa, J. (1971) Reaction of bone to mechanical stimuli Part 1: Continuous and intermittent loading of the tibia in the rabbit. *Folia Morphologica*, **19**, 290–300.

Jones, H.H., Priest, J.D., Hayes, W.C., Tichenor, C.C. and Nagel, D.A. (1977) Humeral hypertrophy in response to exercise. *J. Bone Jt. Surg.*, **59-A**, 204–8.

Kenwright, J. and Goodship, A.E. (1989) Mechanical stimulation of tibial fractures. *Clin. Orthop.*, **241**, 36–47.

Kenwright, J., Goodship, A.E., Kelly, D.J., Newman, J.H., Harris, J.D., Richardson, J.B., Evans, M., Spriggins, A.J., Burrough, S.J. and Rowley, D.I. (1986) Effect of controlled axial movement upon the healing of tibial fractures. *Lancet*, **2**, 1185–7.

Lanyon, L.E. (1972) *In vivo* bone strain recorded from thoracic vertebrae in sheep. *J. Biomech.*, **5**, 277–81.

Lanyon, L.E. (1974) Experimental support for trajectorial theory of bone structure. *J. Bone Jt. Surg.*, **56-B** (1), 160–6.

Lanyon, L.E. (1987) Functional strain in bone tissue as an objective and controlling stimulus for adaptive bone remodelling. *J. Biomech.*, **20**, 1083–93.

Lanyon, L.E., Hampson, W.G.J., Goodship, A.E. and Shah, J.S. (1975) Bone deformation recorded *in vivo* from strain gauges attached to the human tibial shaft. *Acta Orthop. Scand.*, **46**, 256–68.

Lanyon, L.E., Paul, I.L., Rubin, C.T., Thrasher, E.L., Delaura, R., Rose, R.M. and Radin, E.L. (1981) *In vivo* strain measurements from bone and prosthesis following total hip replacement. *J. Bone Jt. Surg.*, **63-A**, 989–1001.

Lanyon, L.E. and Rubin, C.T. (1984) Static versus dynamic loads as an influence on bone remodelling. *J. Biomech.*, **15**, 141–54.

Lanyon, L.E. and Smith, R.N. (1969) Measurements of bone strain in the walking animal. *Res. Vet. Sci.*, **10**, 93–4.

Lanyon, L.E. and Smith, R.N. (1970) Bone strain in the tibia during normal quadrupedal locomotion. *Acta Orthop. Scand.*, **41**, 238–48.

Pope, M.H. and Evans, M. (1982) Design considerations in external fixation, in *Concepts in External Fixation* (eds D. Seligson and M.H. Pope), Grune and Stratton, New York.

Rubin, C.T. (1982) Dynamic strain similarity. PhD thesis, University of Bristol.

Rubin, C.T. and Lanyon, L.E. (1982) Limb mechanics as a function of speed and gait: A study of the functional strains in the radius and tibia of the horse and dog. *J. Exptl. Biol.*, **101**, 187–211.

Rubin, C.T. and Lanyon, L.E. (1984) Dynamical strain similarity in vertebrates: an alternative to allometric limb bone scaling. *J. Theoret. Biol.*, **107**, 321–7.

Rubin, C.T. and Lanyon, L.E. (1987) Osteoregulatory nature of mechanical stimuli: function as a determinant for adaptive remodelling in bone. *J. Orthop. Res.*, **5**, 300–10.

Skerry, T.M., Bitemsky, L., Chayen, J. and Lanyon, L.E. (1988) Loading related reorientation of bone proteoglycans *in vivo*. Strain memory in bone tissue? *J. Orth. Res.*, **6**, 547–51.

Skerry, T.M., Suswillo, R., El Haj, A.J., Ali, N.N., Dodds, R.A. and Lanyon, L.E. (1990) Load induced proteoglycan in bone tissue *in vivo* and *in vitro*. *Calcif. Tiss. Int.*, **46**, 318–26.

Stupakov, G.P., Kazekin, V.S., Koslovsky, A.P. and Korolev, V.V. (1984) Evaluation of changes in human axial skeletal bone structures during long term spaceflights. *Kosmicheskaya Biologica I Aviakosmicheskaya Meditsina*, **18** (2), 33–7.

Wolff, J. (1892) *Das gesetz der transformation der knochen*, von August Hirschwald, Berlin (as translated by Maquet, P. and Furlong, R. (1986) *The Law of Bone Remodelling*, Springer-Verlag, Berlin).

Woo, S.L.-Y., Lothringer, K.S., Akeson, W.J., Coutts, R.D., Wood, Y.K., Simon, B.R. and Gomez, M.A. (1984) Less rigid internal fixation plates: historical prospectives and current concepts. *J. Orthop. Res.*, **1**, 431.

6

Strain telemetry in orthopaedics

A.J.C. Lee, S.J. Taylor and N. Donaldson

6.1 INTRODUCTION

The accuracy with which the stresses in a complex engineering structure can be determined is limited by the accuracy of the estimation of the forces, geometry and constraints applied to the structure. In the field of biomechanics as applied to the human patient, it is often extremely difficult to determine these variables. In consequence, the direct measurement of internal forces or deflections in an implant system using strain gauges and telemetry is of importance, enabling such devices to be designed with much greater confidence than hitherto. This chapter will present a review of the applications of telemetry in orthopaedics to illustrate the range of applications to which it can be applied, the type of data that can be obtained and an overview of modern telemetry techniques.

6.2 APPLICATIONS IN ORTHOPAEDICS

6.2.1 The hip joint

The first report of the use of an instrumented implant at the hip joint is by Rydell (1966). He used a modified Austin Moore hemi-arthroplasty in which the head and neck were hollow, with strain gauges placed on the inside of the neck. Four half bridge circuits were used to determine the moments and two gauges placed in series were used to determine the axial force in the neck. Strain gauge leads were taken out of the implant between the neck and head and led to a connector that was initially left buried under the skin of the patient. Two patients were fitted with measuring prostheses, the first was a 51 year old male who suffered a fracture of the head of the femur in a motor car accident and the second, a 56 year old female who fell and fractured her left femoral neck. Both patients were allowed to recover for 6 months after their operations before the connectors were exposed by a small incision in the skin and connected to the recording apparatus. Recordings were carried out over periods of 6 and 8 days, after which the wires were pulled out of the patients, disconnecting (by breakage) at the join between implant and wires. A number of tests were carried out on both patients, giving the results shown in Table 6.1 ($\times$ body weights).

Table 6.1 Loads recorded for various activities ($\times$ body weight)

	Case 1	*Case 2*
One leg support	2.3	2.8
Level walking (slow)	1.59 (max)	2.95 (max)
Level walking (fast)	1.80 (max)	3.27 (max)
Stair climbing	1.54 (max)	3.38 (max)
Running	Not done	4.33 (max)

English and Kilvington (1979), and Kilvington and Goodman (1981) were the first to report the clinical use of a telemetry system with an implanted data transmitter. One patient was reported, a 59 year old female who underwent left total hip replacement for severe osteoarthritis. Strain gauges were attached to the neck of the femoral stem of an English total hip replacement. Leads from the gauges were led to an encapsulated, battery powered, transmitter that was buried in the fat layer below the skin of the patient. Data from the measuring implant were recorded at operation and for a further 42 days afterwards. Results are shown in Table 6.2. It is unfortunate that English died before the three further planned implantations could be carried out.

Table 6.2 Loads recorded for various activities ($\times$ body weight)

Days post-op	3	4	12	42
Standing	1.20	–	2.42	–
Walking	–	1.85	2.56	2.70
One leg stance	–	–	3.59	–

A rather different type of measuring implant has been designed by Mann and others (Carlson, 1971; Carlson *et al.*, 1974a, b; Hodge *et al.*, 1989) and inserted in one patient providing readings over a period of 5 years before the patient died from unrelated causes. The implant was a modified Moore-type endoprosthesis inserted into a 73 year old female who had sustained a displaced fracture of the femoral head. The head of the implant was modified to accommodate 14 pressure transducers which monitored the contact pressure at the implant–cartilage interface. Ten of the transducers had linear calibration curves for temperature and pressure, four transducers did not meet specifications and were excluded from the quoted results. Pressures during many types of activity were reported: typical maximum pressures were as shown in Table 6.3.

Table 6.3

	Pressure (MPa)
Unsupported walking	5.5
Stair climbing	10.2
Rising from a chair	15.0
Jogging	7.7
Jumping	7.3

The rate of change of pressure at the hip during rising from a chair increased steadily as time went by: from 24 MPas^{-1} at 2 weeks post operation to 107 MPas^{-1} at 1.5 years post operation. Each particular activity produced a peak level of maximum contact pressure in the hip that subsequently decreased and stabilized. For example, the peak occurred 6 months after the operation for walking and 1 year after the operation for stair climbing and rising from a chair. An interesting observation was that the patient seemed to be contracting the hip prior to heel strike – pressures in the hip were observed to lead the force plate recordings (Mann and Hodge, 1990).

In an attempt to measure the strains along the stem of an implanted hip joint stem, Barlow and co-workers (Barlow *et al.*, 1984a, b; Lee, 1986) designed a multi-channel data acquisition telemetry system comprising 15 semiconductor strain gauge channels able to measure strain from −2000 to +1570 microstrain with an overall accuracy of better than 5%. The implanted telemetry used thick-film hybrid technology with circuits mounted on alumina substrates. The first substrate formed the base of a hermetically sealed box containing components which were not themselves hermetically sealed, the second substrate (mounted on top of the first) contained components which had their own hermetic sealing, and a top substrate supported the power receiving and data transmitting coils. The final inter-wired assembly was encapsulated in silicon rubber and connected to the strain gauges on the femoral stem by flexible leads consisting of coiled coils of four wires surrounded by silicone rubber. The external system consisted of the power driver, the logic circuits, 64K RAM pack and computer interface. On completion of data acquisition, the RAM pack was connected to the computer by the interface to facilitate data processing. The whole system was tested in the laboratory only and was shown to function well. However, the overall size of the implanted packages together with the unsolved problem of how to prevent water ingress causing failure of the relatively unprotected gauges meant that the system has not been used in animals or human patients.

Davy and co-workers (1988) have reported on an implanted tele-meterized total hip prosthesis in one patient capable of measuring three mutually perpendicular components of force applied to the femoral head. Power was provided to the implanted circuitry by a pacemaker-type battery that could be turned on/off by a reed switch activated by an external magnet. Output from the three sets of gauges, plus a reference signal, was combined into a single transmitted frequency modulated signal. Usable data were obtained from the implant over seven sessions in 31 days. At 45 days no signal was obtained from the system. Results obtained were as shown in Table 6.4.

Table 6.4

	Maximum resultant force ($\times$ body weight)			
	3 days	6 days	16 days	31 days
Straight leg raise	–	1.0	1.5	1.8
Getting out of bed	0.8	1.0	1.2	1.4
Getting into bed	0.8	1.0	1.5	1.5
Double leg stance	0.5	0.7	0.9	1.0
Single leg stance	1.2	1.3	1.4	2.1
Walking, with aid	1.0	1.5	2.6	2.4, 2.8

A second implant has recently been inserted into a 72 year old male (Davy *et al.*, 1990). Initial results are reported in Table 6.5. Telemetry and force plate/gait measurements were taken at the same time. It was concluded that hip force duration is longer than might be predicted from force plate measurements, that telemeterized implants provide measurements that cannot be predicted from force plate measurements and that current state-of-the-art electronics means that it is now possible to do much more than was possible just a year or two ago.

Table 6.5

	Maximum resultant force ($\times$ body weight)
Walking at 0.9 m/s	2.5
Walking at 1.9 m/s	3.7
Stair climbing	2.5
Rising from a chair	1.2

Two clinically successful long term telemeterized total hip prostheses have been reported widely by Bergmann and co-workers (Bergmann *et al.*, 1988, 1989a, b, c, 1990b, c, d, e; Graichen, 1990). In May and August 1988, instrumented total hip prostheses were implanted in both hips of an 82 year old male with osteoarthritis. Measurements were made from 1 day after the operation. A number of variables were investigated and the following was reported:

(a)   Soft shoes or walking on soft ground do not reduce maximum joint forces during normal activity. Impact forces on the hips are extremely small and depend more on how the patient steps on the ground than the nature of the ground itself or the shoes worn by the patient.

(b)   Passive movement of the patient's leg by a physiotherapist produced small hip joint forces. Active exercises or working against resistance provided by the physiotherapist created forces nearly as high as unsupported walking. A single crutch can be expected to reduce forces to 80–85% of normal values, two crutches may be expected to reduce forces to 60–70% of normal values.

(c)   Standing symmetrically on both legs produces forces between 60% and 130% BW (Body Weight). Standing on one leg produces forces between 270% and 315% BW. Walking at 1–4 km/h produces peak forces between 240% and 355% BW. Jogging at about 6 km/h produces forces between 475% and 550% BW. The strong influence of speed of walking on peak hip joint force reported by Paul (1967) and Röhrle *et al.* (1984) could not be confirmed.

(d)   The relationship between measured hip joint forces and those predicted from force plate measurements was not good.

Taylor and Donaldson (1990) have reported on a telemetry system designed to monitor load transmission in massive implants intended to replace the hip and part of the femur following tumour surgery. Two implant systems are now proposed: implant system Mk I will monitor axial strains at the tip of the implant inside the femoral medullary canal, and in the body of the prosthesis below the neck; and implant system Mk II will, additionally, monitor axial loading and bending at the plateau where the implant bears on the cut surface of the mid-diaphysis of the femur and will monitor axial loading, bending and torsion at several cross-sections along the length of the intramedullary stem. The implanted instrumentation for both systems, fabricated using thick-film technology, is powered inductively via a small implant coil coupled to an external leg coil. Measurements are telemetered from the implant, via the same link. The Mk I system uses metal foil strain gauges and the first device has been implanted recently. Thin film strain gauges are being considered for the Mk II system which is currently under development, as these have superior characteristics to foil gauges in regard to drift over long periods.

Granjon *et al.* (1990) have designed a telemetry system to measure the strains at the interface between hip implant and bone. A cementless femoral stem implant has been designed with a lithium battery powered, hybrid circuit transmitter set in the stem of the implant below the collar. It is connected to a stool hook sensor that is pressed through the cortex of the femur so that the four points of the stool hook rest at the implant/bone interface. Strain of the stool hook is produced by interface movement and transmitted out of the patient via an antenna set around the neck of the stem. The energy needed for the circuits is reported as 100 mW giving an anticipated life of 10 years using a reed relay switch activated externally by a magnet. Unresolved problems are reported with the calibration of the device. In the long term it is intended to replace the batteries with a power receiving coil.

6.2.2 The spine

A number of workers have designed and used telemetry systems for measuring loads carried by various spinal implants. Nachemson and Elfstrom (Nachemson and Elfstrom, 1971; Elfstrom and Nachemson, 1973) have designed a telemetry system for measuring force in Harrington distraction rods used in the treatment of patients with idiopathic scoliosis. At the time of the investigation described in the papers a two stage procedure was used in the treatment of scoliosis in Sweden. The first stage consisted of a release of ligamentous soft tissue around the spine using Harrington rods for distraction. Two weeks later a fusion was performed. In consequence of this two stage technique, Nachemson was able to implant a telemeterized Harrington rod to monitor the loads between the first and second procedures. The method gave important information about the immediate postoperative loading on the rods but the nature of the rather bulky implant required that it be removed at the second stage of the procedure after a very short time of implantation.

Nagel *et al.* (1986) have developed another Harrington rod telemetry system using Kulite semiconductor strain gauges. The gauges were attached to the surface of the distraction rods and covered with an epoxy seal. The gauges were connected to an implanted amplifier, modulator and transmitter. The power was received by an implanted telemetric power supply with externally monitored switching on and automatic switching off after 15 min transmission. A total of seven implants in sheep were reported: the telemetry systems of transmitter, modulator and on/off switches worked perfectly, however the semiconductor strain gauges did not function as well as the telemetry. Problems were reported with breakage of the fine gold leads to the strain gauges and with water seepage between the rods and the gauges. It was reported that further developments would incorporate strain gauges that were hermetically sealed by plasma welding the ends of a thin sleeve placed over the installed gauges.

Crawford *et al.* (1990) reported on telemetry on a Hartshill rectangle spinal fixation implant system. The system was originally designed to answer the following questions: how much spine needs to be supported, how strong should the implant be and for how long should it be applied. A considerable amount of laboratory testing was carried out to develop the telemetry system, in particular, to identify the best sealant to prevent ingress of moisture between gauge and metal. The best coating was reported as successive layers of Ciba Geigy epoxies CY1300 and 753, and Union Carbide Paralene. Implantations were made into two sheep and signals received from the telemetry system. The signals were not such that the progress of fusion could be monitored. A recent development of the system incorporating more sophisticated telemetry packaged in a pacemaker can is currently implanted onto the spine of a baboon and is measuring flexion and torque.

Rohlmann *et al.* (1990) reported on a prototype instrumented internal fixator used for stabilization of fractured vertebrae. The telemetry device uses a modification of the system used in the total hip developed by the group (Bergmann *et al.*, 1988; 1989a, b, c; 1990b, c, d, e, Graichen, 1990), and is designed to measure loads and moments in the implant rods. The internal fixator used is a modified Dick system, comprising sets of two Schanz screws connected by the instrumented rod. The telemetry uses a new, inductively powered eight channel system, with the induction coil strapped to the patient's back. The first implantation is expected in 1991, with a programme calling for about ten implantations.

6.2.3 Bone nails

Nail plate telemetry implantations have been reported by Brown *et al.* (1982) and by Burny *et al.* (1990). Brown and co-workers describe the design and use of a two channel telemeterized nail plate capable of transmitting information on the bending moment developed about the junction of plate and nail. Five nails were implanted of which three produced clinically significant results. All results showed a cyclic pattern of moment, with peak moments of up to 35 N m vertically and 12 N m horizontally being recorded. Burny and co-workers presented their experience using measuring nails as a routine clinical procedure. They were able to report 3 weeks to 3 months direct output from strain gauges mounted on the plate of a fixed blade nail plate. Signals from the gauges mounted on the plates were taken out of the patients with hard wiring. No problems were reported with the penetration of the skin by the signal wires and no special prior consent to the procedure was reported as necessary. Over 250 instrumented plates had been used and the measuring plate was now considered as a safe, routine clinical procedure. The progress of fracture healing could not be monitored effectively with the devices and it was stated that it was difficult to relate X-ray appearance with strain gauge output. A development to attach the system to sliding blade nail plates was reported to be underway.

A telemeterized intramedullary nail has been described by Schneider *et al.* (1990). The requirements of their system were: inductive powering; ability to measure six components of load; measurements to be taken in the region of the defect; large strain range; long term (2 years) stability; telemetric data transmission. The first system described uses an AO/ASIF nail cut into two components with the strain gauges inserted into the nail. Eight channels of strain data could be made available. Measurements of bending, torsion and axial load were obtained as given in Table 6.6. A second system with fifteen channels has been designed but results were not reported.

Table 6.6

Time	18 days PO	182 days PO
Axial torque (N m)	−10	−2
Flexion/extension (N m)	11	2
Abduction/adduction (N m)	−17	−1
Axial force (N)	−760	−510

6.3 DEVELOPMENTS IN PROSPECT

The implanted part of the instrumentation generally consists of four blocks: the strain sensors, some signal processing circuitry (amplifiers, filters, A/D convertors, etc.), the telemeter and the power supply. Two or more of these blocks may be combined in the case of an inductively powered system where the inductive link also functions as the telemeter (Taylor and Donaldson, 1990).

The main developments since Rydell (1966), in common with many other fields of measurement, have been in electronics and this has led to improvements in circuit density, performance, complexity and power consumption. Modern implants may be designed with one or more LSI CMOS processing blocks, bi-CMOS low-drift front end amplifiers and a 10–12 bit CMOS analogue-to-digital converter. These integrated circuits may be available as surface mounted parts or as die for chip-and-wire applications, yielding a complex instrumentation system in a very confined space. With access to the right capital equipment, the bioengineer can now design an ASIC (application specific integrated circuit) which embodies on a single chip most of the amplifiers, multiplexers, A/D converters, filters, and all the digital processing required prior to telemetry. Analogue and digital functions can be integrated (with possible compromise in analogue performance) and the miniaturization available especially in die form means that instrumentation can be placed close to sensors, eliminating crosstalk and electromagnetic pickup. One way in which this may be beneficial in multi-sensor applications is that an ASIC could be placed at each sensor site, connected to other remote sites and to the telemeter using a 1- or 2-wire bus, with which each site is interrogated and data transmitted. With a proven ASIC design such a method may improve reliability by reducing the number of wires and enabling easier construction.

Implant power supplies have used batteries and implanted switches (Berilla *et al.*, 1990), or induction of power either at radiofrequency (Taylor and Donaldson, 1990; Mann and Burgess, 1990) or audiofrequency (Bergmann *et al.*, 1990a). Inductive supplies are generally preferred, although power must be kept at tolerable levels for national regulations, pickup by the instrumentation or sensor leads, and tissue temperature. The choice of inductive link design depends on the desired or acceptable location of the implanted coil. If this is constrained to lie inside the prosthesis, Graichen (1990) has shown that a magnetic concentrating material made from a high permittivity alloy can be used to increase the induction at the implant, but this is only effective at audio frequencies (Bergmann *et al.*, 1990a). Nevertheless, efficiency is still poor, requiring a large magnetic field and an implant circuit that demands little power. With this arrangement, however, everything is contained within the prosthesis, and possible biocompatibility problems are avoided. If the implant coil is positioned outside the prosthesis, power transfer efficiency is greatly improved (Taylor and Donaldson, 1990). Furthermore, radio frequencies may be used for powering, which allows a small coil to be used with a ferrite core and requires only a small tuning capacitor. The use of RF also allows telemetry at useful data rates using passive signalling (Donaldson, 1986). The design of inductively powered systems is not a well defined art, and several compromises must generally be made with regard to efficiency, coil separation insensitivity, etc. (Donaldson and Perkins, 1983). Developments have been made in the design of inductive links for maximizing performance of particular parameters, e.g. coil separation insensitivity (Donaldson, 1987a, b), although this is only applicable for well-coupled coils. Orthopaedic applications usually require a small implant coil which means that the coupling coefficient between implant and external coil is poor (although not strongly dependent on the position of the external coil), and therefore such stratagems cannot usefully be employed. In this situation achieving good efficiency is the overriding consideration.

Data telemetry from an implanted device to a remote receiver either attached to or remote from the patient can be accomplished either using radio transmission or via the inductive link used for powering. Examples of the former (Berilla *et al.*, 1990; Mann and Burgess, 1990; Bergmann *et al.*, 1990a) use FM transmitters at frequencies between 76 and 150 MHz with a variety of pulse modulation techniques. The latter 'passive signalling' technique, referred to above, employs pulse-interval modulation by short circuiting the implant tuned circuit, causing reflected impedance modulation at the energizing coil (Taylor and Donaldson, 1990).

It would seem that the area which has seen least change since Rydell (1966) is the strain sensor. Metal foil and semiconductor strain gauges have been used exclusively in orthopaedic strain measurements, due to their good availability and ease of application although it is widely acknowledged that they usually have poor long-term stability, an important factor in applications where no recalibration is possible, as is usually the case with implanted devices. Temperature coefficients may also be poor, although usually minimized by proper choice of foil gauge. These effects may be ameliorated by having a Wheatstone Bridge for each signal (Davy *et al.*, 1990) which will correct for temperature and, partially, for drift. The total number of gauges can be reduced however if, following Bergmann *et al.* (1982), only one gauge per unknown variable is employed and the 'Matrix Method' is used to extract the variables from the strain signals. This facilitates construction of the device but requires more stable strain sensors. Despite improvements in all other aspects of telemetry systems, the unknowns due to sensor inaccuracies remain. It is here that the greatest challenge exists for improvement in measurement accuracy.

6.3.1 Major prostheses with internal gauges

Several workers have reported results with foil and semiconductor gauges which have been mounted inside a cavity which provides them with a hermetic seal. These include hip prostheses where the aim has been to measure either the forces acting on the neck (Bergmann *et al.*, 1990e; Davy *et al.*, 1990) or the pressures on the head during articulation (Mann and Burgess, 1990). In two of these prostheses (Mann and Burgess, 1990; Bergmann *et al.*, 1990a) the cavity is welded, and in the other (Davy *et al.*, 1990) a combination of teflon, epoxy and silicone rubber is used to prevent fluid ingress to the gauges and electronics.

The Boston group (Mann and Burgess, 1990) use semiconductor gauges diffused into the surface of a single crystal silicon cantilever, to measure deflection of a pressure-measuring diaphragm. This appears to avoid the use of epoxy to mount the gauges. It is estimated from the published data that the maximum strain experienced by these gauges for the maximum applied stress of 18 MPa is about 250 microstrain. There was no reference to any reported drift figures for these gauges.

The Berlin group (Bergmann *et al.*, 1990a) also use semiconductor gauges, but attach them to the inside surface of the prosthetic neck with a proprietary adhesive. Maximum expected strains were 850 microstrain. Drift was noticed in the gauges after about 1 year. After 2 years, the offset in the axial component of force was estimated at 60 N and much smaller in the perpendicular directions. Gauge drift could be calculated from the coefficients in the matrix used for force calculation. The authors state that in their opinion the drift would have been much more severe had foil gauges been used instead of semiconductor gauges. The Cleveland, Ohio group (Davy *et al.*, 1990) also use semiconductor gauges attached to the inside of the prosthetic neck with adhesive. There did not appear to be any reference to the levels of strain being measured or any estimation of drift. Semiconductor gauges offer a very useful improvement in gauge factor, typically 70 times that of foil gauges. However, they have large temperature coefficients, and are more difficult to place than foil gauges.

For any strain gauge, if the zero drift rate is significant compared to the required resolution and dynamic range, the signal will soon become doubtful. From results of work carried out by two of the authors (ST and ND) to measure drift of foil gauges on titanium, reported below, it appears that for long-term strain measurements even dry gauges experiencing strain may have significant drift. For dry gauges at a constant strain of 2000 microstrain it was found that drift rates as high as 0.7 microstrain/day continued for over 130 days. Although unstrained dry gauges showed no net drift, the rate of drift at intermediate rates of applied strain was not investigated. It was concluded that the drift was probably related to the stresses locked up in the adhesive used to bond the gauge to the substrate, although there is insufficient evidence to be sure about this. Scepticism therefore about the stability of gauges (both foil and semiconductor) which use an adhesive led to the investigation of other types of strain sensor.

Alternative types of strain gauge may be made by depositing thin or thick films. Thin films (Hopewell, 1972) are deposited by sputtering an insulator (typically silica or borosilicate), followed by nichrome or other suitable conductor onto a finely polished flat metal surface. The gauge pattern is defined by photolithography or laser cutting, which give tight tolerances on the unstrained resistance values (0.1%). Ideally the gauges will be deposited directly onto the prosthesis so that there is no drift due to the bonding between the substrate which bears the gauges and the prosthesis itself, as there is for foil and semiconductor gauges. The conductor being metallic, gauge factors are similar to foil gauges (about 2). The major advantage is their stability: zero drift of 0.02% of full range per year, and creep of 0.03% after 20×10^6 cycles to full range are feasible. However, it may need years of experience to become confident of achieving this performance and a good deal of capital equipment is required. For these reasons, fabrication of the gauges will usually be best done by a specialist company (e.g. Strain Measurement Devices Ltd, Sharon Road, Bury St Edmunds, UK).

An attraction of thick film gauges is that the technology is much cheaper than thin film and is, therefore, more practicable in the laboratory. The gauges are formed by screen printing layers of resistive and conductive pastes onto an insulating substrate and firing each print at a temperature of 600–1000°C, depending on the paste composition, to sinter the particles. The geometry of the gauge can be designed for the application. Gauge factors (GF) vary from 2 to 18, depending on the resistor paste (Catteneo *et al.*, 1980). On balance, the low GF pastes are to be preferred because their transverse sensitivity is lower (Morten *et al.*, 1979) and because the drift, expressed in microstrain per year, is lower (Dell'Acqua *et al.*, 1982; Coleman, 1984). If screen printing facilities are available in the laboratory, for example for producing thick-film hybrid circuits, these gauges may be produced easily, and become especially attractive in quantity. Resistance tolerance is generally poor, unless laser trimming is used and Temperature Coefficient of Resistance (TCR) figures vary between 10 and 400 ppm/°C depending upon the resistor paste. These figures are for resistors on alumina, which is the normal substrate for this technology. To take advantage of this type of gauge, the substrate must be bonded to the prosthesis by a technique which does not allow creep. Leaving aside polymeric adhesives, two possible methods are as follows. One could take advantage of the high temperature tolerance of thick films and braze the alumina to the prosthesis. Because the thermal expansion coefficients of alumina and (for example) titanium are not very dissimilar (7.0 and 9.6 ppm/°C respectively), the residual stresses might not be significant. Alternatively, instead of an alumina substrate, the gauges could be printed onto a metallic substrate with a glass or ceramic coating (e.g. Jones, 1985) and the metal could then be welded to the prosthesis. These are untried possibilities. Some such technique must be shown to give good drift performance in this application before thick film strain gauges can be said to perform better than adhesive-bonded types.

An entirely different type of strain sensor is the vibrating beam whose natural frequency depends on the applied strain. Beams must be designed to have small energy losses so that their Qs are high; most commonly a double-ended tuning fork arrangement is used (EerNisse and Paros, 1983; Haroda *et al.*, 1986; Cheshmehdoost, 1989), though single beams are possible (US Patent 3470400: Single beam force transducer with integral mounting isolation) as is planar construction with photolithographic definition (US Patent 4372173: Resonator force transducer). Pickup and drive transducers are required to provide positive feedback to maintain oscillation at resonance. This can be accomplished piezoelectrically (Haroda *et al.*, 1986) or using electro-magnetic drive and optical pickup (Halliwell, 1987). The advantages of using transducers of this kind are: large strain sensitivity (typically 150–300 times that of foil gauges), very low power consumption, and that the output parameter is frequency rather than a small analogue voltage. This latter property means that an entire telemetry system could be operated in the digital domain, avoiding the need for stable high-gain amplifiers. In applications where it is desirable to realize the system using a custom IC, for example in implanted applications where space is at a premium, exclusively digital circuitry is easier and cheaper to implement reliably than mixed analogue and digital functions. Two of the authors (ST and ND) made a double-ended tuning fork but found it was very sensitive to off axis loading: its sensitivity to shear force, applied between its ends, was about ten times higher than to axial force (EerNisse and Paros, 1983). Unfortunately this could not be corrected by a calibration matrix (with more than one sensor in use) because the frequency–strain response was also non-linear. It seems, therefore, that the beams must be mounted in such a way that they are only subject to the axial component of strain. If this is to be made small enough to rival a strain gauge for use in prostheses, developments in micromachining to yield a beam or beams with mount-ing, all in a single crystal of silicon, should be watched. The question of how to bond this to the prosthesis remains.

These five types of strain sensor are compared in Table 6.7.

6.3.2 Prostheses with external gauges

Some prostheses are too small to enclose a cavity or it is impractical or undesirable to make them hollow: these must have their gauges on the external surface of the load-bearing member. The gauges and the joints to their connecting wires must then be protected from the body fluids by an encapsulant. Several devices of this type have been described (Walmsley *et al.*, 1978; Burny *et al.*, 1990; Lee and Barlow, 1990; Granjon *et al.*, 1990) but their working lives have been short and it is no doubt significant that little has been written about how the

Table 6.7 Strain sensors; comparison of various types of gauges and vibrating beams

	Sensitivity (gauge factor)	*Temperature coefficient*	*Unstrained drift rate*
Foil	2.1	Material selected to minimize thermal effects (Measurements Group, 1983)	20 microstrain/year (with practice) (Freynik *et al.*, 1976)
Semiconductor*	Up to 200	Up to 10 000 ppm/°C	
Thin film†	1.9	20 ppm/°C	< 0.02% of full scale per year
Thick film (on alumina)	2–50 (Cattaneo *et al.*, 1980)	10 to 400 ppm/°C (Cattaneo *et al.*, 1980)	Approx. 2 microstrain per year
Vibrating beam (Elinvar Alloy) (Haroda *et al.*, 1986)	700	3 ppm/°C (deduced)	0.03 microstrain per 1000 h at 50°C (deduced)

* Strain Gauges, Kulite Sensors Limited, Marbaix House, Besemer Road, Basingstoke, RG21 3LG, UK.
† Strain Measurement Devices Limited, Sharon Road, Bury St. Edmunds, IP33 3TZ, UK.

encapsulants were chosen though the authors sometimes record that the encapsulant ought to be a good barrier to body fluid. Crawford *et al.* (1990) have tested a wide range of candidate materials but found none which were satisfactory for chronic use, judged by the stability of the strain signals and the insulation resistance to the prosthesis.

A similar search, through a diverse selection of polymers, for a material to protect the circuits of neurological prostheses was made 20 years ago (Donaldson, 1973, 1987c) while the desirable properties for the encapsulants for integrated circuits was given by White as long ago as 1969 (White, 1969). This work established that highly permeable materials can be good encapsulants and therefore that encapsulants should not be regarded as water vapour barriers. This is fortunate because the range of permeability for polymers covers about three orders of magnitude (Traeger, 1977) and the vapour takes only hours to approach equilibrium in a coating of the most permeable materials (Troyk *et al.*, 1986) so it is impossible, with any polymer, to exclude the vapour for the years needed for a chronic implant. The encapsulant works by occupying the surface between the conductors (there must be no bubbles or regions without adhesion) so that although the polymer will be saturated with vapour, there are no voids into which liquid can condense. For it is liquid, even if pure water, which causes failure by carrying ionic leakage currents (which in this case will shunt the gauge giving a lower apparent resistance), and by allowing corrosion of the gauge alloy (increasing its resistance). Should the liquid extend to the metal of the prosthesis, the gauge isolation resistance will fall. To occupy the surface, the encapsulant must adhere, and continue to adhere, throughout the required life of the gauge. As maintenance of this adhesion depends both on the strength of the adhesive bond and on the stresses to which it is subject, it is desirable that the material should have low modulus so that strains in the material, due to temperature or humidity changes, do not cause large stresses. Surface cleanliness prior to encapsulation is of great importance as it will affect the adhesion but also, should there be some liquid at the interface, the ionic content and thus the corrosiveness and osmolality of the solution. The concentration of solutes also depends on the amount of ionizable matter in the encapsulant itself.

Many silicone rubbers and gels have been found to be satisfactory for the protection of integrated circuits: there is substantial literature. Neurological prostheses, which are like instrumented orthopaedic prostheses in that they operate in the body, can use silicones alone to protect their electronics. This approach is now seen to be so successful that high reliability integrated circuits may soon be encapsulated in this way instead of enclosing them inside gas-filled hermetic packages (which are water vapour barriers) (Balde, 1989). Such a change in the electronics industry will require greater understanding (Sinnadurai, 1981; Wong *et al.*, 1989) and further dissemination of good encapsulation practice. For metal strain gauges passing a current of about 1 mA, measurement to an accuracy of 1 ppm (i.e. about 0.5 microstrain) requires that the leakage currents remain less than 1 nA: for some combinations of substrate and encapsulant, this has been shown to be possible (Sbar and Kozakiewicz, 1978; Troyk, *et al.* 1986). On this evidence, it seems probable that strain gauges on the external surfaces of prostheses could be insulated sufficiently well for failures due to leakage and corrosion to be prevented. However, unlike the other types of film device mentioned, strain gauges may suffer from another unfavourable effect of water vapour: the insulating layer or layers between the resistive element and the prosthesis may creep at a rate which is strongly affected by vapour pressure. For foil gauges, bonded by the recommended proprietary adhesive, the supplier asked was unable to give any information about the effect of humidity. The only reference which bears on this topic (Hughes *et al.*, 1984) shows that another commercial unfilled epoxy has a creep rate which increases very quickly with rising relative humidity. The authors (ST and ND) have carried out a test to compare the drift rate of foil gauges on titanium, either kept 'dry' by silica gel or at 77% RH (within an encapsulant *in vivo* the humidity would be 100%). It was found that while the unstrained dry samples had negligible average drift, the three in damper air drifted at up to 0.5 microstrain per day until their environment was made dry when they too stopped drifting. Unfortunately, it was not possible to confirm that this effect was due to creep in the adhesive rather than corrosion of the gauge alloy. As far as is known, the creep performance of foil gauges at steady high humidity remains largely unknown. Fortunately, this uncertainty can largely be circumvented if thin-film gauges are used instead of foil gauges. Since most glasses absorb relatively little water, it is likely that the excellent creep performance of this type of gauge (see above) will not be much reduced by high humidity. The opinion of the authors is that it should be possible to make highly stable external gauges by sputter-deposition of glass and then a nickel–chrome gauge directly on the prosthesis. After attaching wires, the gauge and the joints would be encapsulated in a soft silicone. This might need to be protected during subsequent handling and movement within soft tissue by some sort of rigid shield, which might be welded or glued so as to cover the gauge site. Its function would however be entirely mechanical. The development of external gauges in this way would require a good deal of laboratory testing. If good drift performance was desired, the tests should be designed to distinguish between drifts due to corrosion, leakage current and creep.

6.4 CONCLUSIONS

Improvements in integrated circuit technology are making it easier to add implantable strain telemetry to prostheses. Power can be provided from a battery or by induction. Part of the information which one would like to obtain from these devices concerns the slow changes which occur as the body and the prosthesis interact in the long term. These changes in loading cause changes in the measured strain which are often small compared to the drift rates of adhesive-bonded strain gauges. For major prostheses, which are made hollow and then hermetically sealed with sensors inside, the drift rates could be reduced by using different types of sensor which need not use adhesive. Of the three candidates discussed, thin film is the most readily available and proven. Thick film gauges can have low drift and are more suitable for production in the small laboratory, but some satisfactory method of bonding substrates to the prosthesis must be found. Vibrating beams are attractive because they dispense with the need for stable amplifiers, but they must be miniaturized with proper mounts and have some means of linearization before they can compete with strain gauges. Progress in the micromachine industry should be watched for this development. When gauges are not hermetically sealed, they must operate at 100% humidity. This requires a good encapsulant and interlayers between the gauges and the prosthesis which will not creep. Thin film gauges under silicone encapsulant look promising and should be tested.

The value of data yielded by telemetry together with the rapid advancements in integrated circuit technology assures the future for such strain measuring systems.

REFERENCES

Balde, J.W. (1989) The IEEE Gel Task Force: An early look at final testing. *IEEE Trans. Compon., Hybrids Manufact. Technol.*, **12**, 426–9.

Barlow, J.W., Goldie, I.F., Horwood, J.M.K., Lee, A.J.C. and Ransom, R.P. (1984a) *In vivo* telemetry of strain in a total hip joint. *Proc. Conf. on Engineering and Clinical Aspects of Endo-prosthetic Fixation*, Paper C216/84, Institute of Mechanical Engineers, London, pp. 55–62.

Barlow, J.W., Horwood, J.M.K., Lee, A.J.C. and Ransome, R.P. (1984b) A thick film implantable data acquisition module. *Proc. Internepcon-UK*, pp. 367–74.

Bergmann, G., Graichen, F. and Rohlmann, A. (1989a) Five months *in-vivo* measurement of hip joint forces. *Trans. XII Int. Congr. of Biomech.*, Los Angeles, Int. Society of Biomechanics, paper no. 43.

Bergmann, G., Graichen, F. and Rohlmann, A. (1989b) Load directions at hip prostheses measured *in-vivo*. *Trans. XII Int. Congr. of Biomech.*, Los Angeles, paper no. 44.

Bergmann, G., Rohlmann, A. and Graichen, F. (1989c) *In-vivo* messung der Huftgelenkbelastung. 1. Teil: Krankengymnastik. *Z. Orthop.*, **127**, 672–79.

Bergmann, G., Rohlmann, A. and Graichen, F. (1990d) Hip joint forces during physical therapy after joint replacement. *Trans. 36th annual ORS meeting*, New Orleans.

Bergmann, G., Rohlmann, A. and Graichen, F. (1990e) *In-vivo* hip joint force measurements in one patient, in *Clinical Implant Materials* (eds G. Heimke, U. Soltész and A.J.C. Lee), Elsevier Science Publisher, B.V., Amsterdam, pp. 639–44.

Bergmann, G., Graichen, F. and Rohlmann, A. (1990a) Instrumentation of a hip joint prosthesis, in *Implantable Telemetry in Orthopaedics* (eds G. Bergmann, F. Graichen and A. Rohlmann), Forshungsvermillung der FU, Berlin, pp. 35–63.

Bergmann, G., Neff, G., Rohlmann, A. and Graichen, F. (1990c) Influence of orthotic devices on the forces at the hip joint. *Trans. 36th annual ORS meeting*, New Orleans.

Bergmann, G., Siraky, J., Rohlmann, A. and Kölbel, R. (1982) Measurement of spatial forces by the 'Matrix' method. *Proc. V/VI 9th World Congress IMECO*, Berlin, pp. 395–404.

Bergmann, G., Graichen, F., Siraky, J., Jendrzynski, H. and Rohlmann, A. (1988) Multichannel strain gauge telemetry for orthopaedic implants. *J. Biomech.*, **21** (2), 169–76.

Bergmann, G., Kniggendorf, H., Rohlmann, A., Graichen, F. and Jendrzynski,

H. (1990b) The influence of floor materials and shoes on the hip joint loading. *Trans. Eur. Soc. Biomech.*, Aarhus, Denmark, B40.

Berilla, J., Davy, D.T., Oyen, O.J. and Heiple, K.G. (1990) Design and fabrication of a multi-channel strain gauge telemetry system, in *Implantable Telemetry in Orthopaedics* (eds G. Bergmann, F. Graichen and A. Rohlmann), Forshungs-vermillung der FU, Berlin, pp. 25–33.

Brown, R.H., Burstein, A.H. and Frankel, V.H. (1982) Telemetering *in vivo* loads from nail plate implants. *J. Biomech.*, **15** (11), 815–23.

Burny, F., Donkerwolcke, M. and Moulart, F. (1990) Monitoring of orthopaedic implants, in *Implantable Telemetry in Orthopaedics* (eds G. Bergmann, F. Graichen and A. Rohlmann), Forshungsvermillung der FU, Berlin, pp. 11–22.

Carlson, C.E. (1971) A proposed method for measuring pressures on the human hip joint. *Exptl. Mech.*, **11** (11), 499–506.

Carlson, C.E., Mann, R.W. and Harris, W.H. (1974a) A radio telemetry device for monitoring cartilage surface pressures in the human hip. *IEEE Trans. Biomed. Engng.*, **21** (4), 257–64.

Carlson, C.E., Mann, R.W. and Harris, W.H. (1974b) A look at the prosthesis–-cartilage interface: design of a hip prosthesis containing pressure transducers. *J. Biomed. Mater. Res.*, **8** (4 Pt 2), 261–9.

Cattaneo, A., Dell'Acqua, R., Dell'Orto, G. and Pirozzi, I. (1980) A practical utilization of the piezoresistive effect in thick film resistors: a low-cost pressure sensor. *Proc. of Microelectronics Symposium*, ISHM, New York, pp. 221.

Chesmehdoost, A. (1989) Double-ended tuning fork theory and design. PhD thesis, Brunel University.

Coleman, M. (1984) Aging mechanisms and stability in thick-film resistors. *Hybrid Circuits*, **4**, 36–41.

Crawford, R.J., Sell, P.J. and Dove, J. (1990) The development of an implantable strain gauge and telemetry system to study *in vivo* loads on a segmental spinal instrumentation implant, in *Implantable Telemetry in Orthopaedics* (eds G. Bergmann, F. Graichen and A. Rohlmann), Forshungsvermillung der FU, Berlin, pp. 137–52.

Davy, D.T., Kotzar, G.M., Berilla, J. and Brown, R.H. (1990) Telemeterized orthopaedic implant work at Case Western Reserve University, in *Implantable Telemetry in Orthopaedics* (eds G. Bergmann, F. Graichen and A. Rohlmann), Forshungsvermillung der FU, Berlin, pp. 205–19.

Davy, D.T., Kotzar, G.M., Brown, R.H., Heiple, K.G., Goldberg, V.M., Heiple, K.G. Jr, Berilla, J. and Berstein, A.H. (1988) Telemetric force measurements across the hip after total arthroplasty. *J. Bone Jt Surg.*, **70A**, 45–50.

Dell'Acqua, R., Dell'Orto, G. and Simonetta, A. (1982) Long term stability of thick-film resistors under strain. *Int. J. Hybrid Microelectr.*, **5**, 82–5.

Donaldson, N. de N. (1986) Passive signalling via inductive coupling. *Med. & Biol. Engng. & Comput.*, **24**, 223–4.

Donaldson, N. and Perkins, T.A. (1983) Analysis of resonant coupled coils in the design of radiofrequency transcutaneous links. *Med. & Biol. Engng. & Comput.*, **21**, 612–27.

Donaldson, P.E.K. (1973) Experimental visual prosthesis. *Proc. IEEE*, **120**, 281–98.

Donaldson, P.E.K. (1987a) Three separation-insensitive radiofrequency inductive links. *J. Med. Engng. & Technol.* **11** (1), 23–9.

Donaldson, P.E.K. (1987b) Power for neurological prostheses: A simple inductive R.F. link with improved performance. *J. Biomed. Engng.*, **9**, 194–7.

Donaldson, P.E.K. (1987c) Twenty years of neurological prostheses-making. *J. Biomed. Engng*, **9**, 291–8.

EerNisse, E.P. and Paros, J.M. (1983) Practical considerations for miniature quartz resonator force transducers. *Proc. of 37th Annual Frequency Control Symposium*, IEEE US Army Electron Res. Dev. Committee, Philadelphia, pp. 255–60.

Elfstrom, G. and Nachemson, A. (1973) Telemetry recordings of forces in the Harrington distraction rod: a method for increasing safety in the operative treatment of scoliosis patients. *Clin. Orthop.*, **93**, 158–72.

English, T.A. and Kilvington, M. (1979) *In vivo* records of hip loads using a femoral stem implant with telemetric output (a preliminary report). *J. Biomed. Engng.*, **1** (2), 111–15.

Freynik, H.S. and Dittbenner, G.R. (1976) Strain gauge stability measurements for years at 75°C in air. *Exptl. Mech.*, **16** (4), 155–60.

Graichen, F. (1990) *Implantierbares telemetrisches ubertragungssystem zur in-vivo-messung belastung kunstlicher huftgelenke*, Schiele & Schon, Berlin, p. 198.

Granjon, Y., Yvroud, E., Mehenni, M. and Abignoli, M. (1990) Biotelemetry for the strain at the interface between hip joint prosthesis and bone: implantation problems, in *Implantable Telemetry in Orthopaedics* (eds G. Bergmann, F. Graichen and A. Rohlmann), Forshungsvermillung der FU, Berlin, pp. 173–7.

Halliwell, M.J. (1987) Pressure transducers using double-ended tuning forks. PhD thesis, University of Manchester Institute of Science and Technology.

Haroda, K., Ikeda, K. and Ueda, T. (1986) Precision transducers using mechanical resonators. *Transduc. Technol.*, **29**, 30.

Hodge, W.A., Carlson, K.L., Fijan, R.S., Burgess, R.G., Riley, P.O., Harris, W.H. and Mann, R.W. (1989) Contact pressures from an instrumented hip endoprosthesis. *J. Bone Jt. Surg.*, **71-A**, 1378–86.

Hopewell, B. (1972) The thin film strain gauge. Lecture delivered at meeting of Stress Analysis Group of the Institute of Physics, The Application of Modern Techniques and Instrumentation in Stress Analysis, 18–20 September 1972 at Royal Military College of Science, Shrivenham, 10 pp.

Hughes, E.J., Routilier, J. and Rutherford, J.L. (1984) The effects of moisture on the dimensional stability of adhesively-bonded joints, in *Adhesive Joints* (ed. K.L. Mittel), Plenum Press, New York, pp. 137–50.

Jones, R.W. (1985) Glass-ceramic coated metal substrates. *Hybrid Circuits*, **6**, 60–1.

Kilvington, M. and Goodman, R.M.F. (1981) *In-vivo* hip joint forces recorded on a strain gauged 'English' prosthesis using an implanted transmitter. *Engng. Med.*, **10** (4), 175–87.

Lee, A.J.C. (1986) *In-vivo* telemetry of total hip joint stresses. *Biomedical Engineering V – Recent Developments. Proc. Fifth Southern Biomedical Engineering Conference* (ed. S. Saha), Pergamon Press, Oxford, pp. 265–8.

Lee, A.J.C. and Barlow, J.W. (1990) The Exeter telemetry system, in *Implantable*

Telemetry in Orthopaedics (eds G. Bergmann, F. Graichen and A. Rohlmann), Forshungsvermillung der FU, Berlin, pp. 77–85.

Mann, R.W. and Burgess, R.G. (1990) An instrumented prosthesis for measuring pressure on acetabular cartilage *in-vivo*, in *Implantable Telemetry in Orthopaedics* (eds G. Bergmann, F. Graichen and A. Rohlmann), Forshungsvermillung der FU, Berlin, pp. 65–75.

Mann, R.W. and Hodge, W.A. (1990) *In vivo* pressures on acetbular cartilage following endoprosthesis surgery, during recovery and rehabilitation, and in the activities of daily living, in *Implantable Telemetry in Orthopaedics* (eds G. Bergmann, F. Graichen and A. Rohlmann), Forshungsvermillung der FU, Berlin, pp. 181–204.

Measurements Group Limited (1983) Temperature-induced apparent strain and gauge factor variation in strain gauges, Tech. Note TN–504.

Morten, B., Pirozzi, L., Prudenziati, M. and Taroni, A. (1979) Strain sensitivity in film and cermet resistors: measured and physical quantities. *Int. J. Hybrid Microelect.*, **12**, L51.

Nachemson, A. and Elfstrom, G. (1971) Intravital wireless telemetry of axial forces in Harrington distraction rods in patients with idiopathic scoliosis. *J. Bone Jt. Surg.*, **53-A**, 445–64.

Nagel, D., Koogle, T., Cordey, J., Frigg, R., Tepic, S., Schlegel, U., Schneider, E. and Perren, S.M. (1986) *In-vivo* measurements of load on Harrington distraction rods in sheep spines with and without fusion. Workshop on human implant telemetry, Rome.

Paul, J.P. (1967) Forces transmitted by joints in the human body. *Proc. I. Mech. E.*, **181**, 8–15.

Rohlmann, A., Bergmann, G. and Graichen, F. (eds) (1990) An instrumented spinal internal fixation device for *in-vivo* load measurements, in *Implantable Telemetry in Orthopaedics*, (eds. G. Bergmann, F. Graichen and A. Rohlmann), Forshungsvermillung der FU, Berlin, pp. 163–72.

Röhrle, H., Scholten, R., Sigolotto, C., Sollbach, W. and Kellner, H. (1984) Joint forces in the human pelvis-leg skeleton during walking. *J. Biomech.*, **17**, 409–24.

Rydell, N.W. (1966) Forces acting on the femoral head–prosthesis. A study on strain gauges supplied prostheses in living persons. *Acta Orthop. Scand., Suppl. 88.*

Sbar, N.L. and Kozakiewicz, R.P. (1978) New acceleration factors for temperature and humidity bias testing. *16th Annual Proc. Reliability Physics*, Symposium IEEE, pp. 161–78.

Schneider, E., Michel, M.C., Genge, M. and Perren, S.M. (1990) Loads acting on an intramedullary femoral nail, in *Implantable Telemetry in Orthopaedics* (eds G. Bergmann, F. Graichen and A. Rohlmann), Forshungsvermillung der FU, Berlin, pp. 221–31.

Sinnadurai, N. (1981) An evaluation of plastic coatings for microcircuits. *ISHM 3rd European Hybrid Microelectronics Conference*, Avignon, pp. 482–495.

Taylor, S. and Donaldson, N. (1990) Instrumenting Stanmore Prostheses for long-term measurement *in-vivo*, in *Implantable Telemetry in Orthopaedics* (eds G. Bergmann, F. Graichen and A. Rohlmann), Forshungsvermillung der FU, Berlin, pp. 93–102.

Traeger, R.K. (1977) Non-hermeticity of polymeric lid sealants. *IEEE Trans. Parts, Hybrids and Packaging*, **13**, 147–52.

Troyk, P.R., Watson, M.J. and Poyezdela, J.J. (1986) Humidity testing of silicone polymers for corrosion control of implanted electronic prostheses, in *Polymeric Materials for Corrosion Control* (eds R.A. Dickie and F.L. Floyd), American Chemical Society Symposium No. 322.

Walmsley, B., Hodgson, J.A. and Burke, R.E. (1978) Forces produced by the medial gastrocnemius and the soleus muscles during locomotion in freely moving cats. *J. Neurophysiol.*, **41**, 1203–8.

White, M.L. (1969) Encapsulation of integrated circuits. *Proc. IEEE*, **57**, 1610–15.

Wong, C.P., Segelken, J.M. and Balde, J.W. (1989) Understanding the use of silicone gels for non-hermetic plastic packaging. *Proc. IEEE*, **12**, 421–5.

7

Two- and three-dimensional photoelastic techniques
J.F. Orr

7.1 INTRODUCTION

The photoelastic technique involves the observation of patterns of dark and light lines, known as fringes, which result from interference of components of plane polarized light when transmitted by a stressed plastic model. This phenomenon was first observed by Brewster early in the 19th century (Frocht, 1941) and subsequently related to stresses in materials. The practical application of the technique increased as suitable modelling materials became available to replace glass, which is optically insensitive and difficult to work. The first such material, 'Celluloid', was used by Coker in 1906 but since then a range of further materials have become available. Applications in biomechanics have been developing since the 1940s.

The experimental examination of photoelastic models (Dally and Riley, 1965; Kuske and Robertson, 1974) is carried out in an instrument known as a polariscope, the main optical elements of which are detailed in Figure 7.1. When plane polarized light is transmitted by a stressed plastic model two groups of dark fringes are visible, called

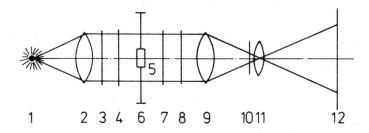

Figure 7.1 Arrangement of a transmission polariscope. 1, Light source; 2, lens; 3, polarizer; 4, quarter wave plate; 5, model; 6, loading frame; 7, quarter wave plate; 8, analyser; 9, lens; 10, filter; 11, projection lens; 12, screen.

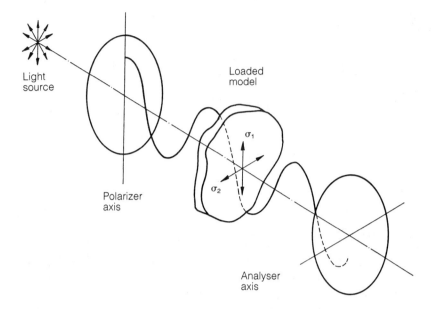

Figure 7.2 Extinction of light to form isoclinic fringe.

isoclinics and *isochromatics*, which give information about directions and magnitudes of principal stresses respectively. The main optical elements, called the polarizer and analyser, each only transmit light along one axis. Thus the plane polarized light which is incident on a model may be considered as a transverse wave lying in a single plane. The polarizer and analyser are normally set with their axes at 90° to each other.

When a two-dimensional plastic model is stressed in the loading frame, the material becomes 'double refracting'. This means that light is transmitted along two perpendicular axes which are aligned in the directions of the principal stresses at any point in the plane of the model. If one of these principal stress directions coincides with the plane of the incident polarized light then the light will be transmitted through the model but will then suffer extinction when it encounters the analyser set out at 90° to the initial plane of polarization, Figure 7.2. Hence dark fringes will result along the loci of all principal stresses whose directions coincide with the polarizer/analyser axes. Other areas of the model will appear light. Rotation of the polarizer and analyser, whilst maintaining the perpendicular relationship of their axes of transmission, allows the loci of principal stresses in all directions to be identified.

The two light waves transmitted at any point of the stressed model not only coincide with the directions of the principal stresses but are transmitted with velocities which are dependent on the stress magnitudes. The transmitted waves will have varying phase relationships as they exit the model which allows constructive and destructive interference and hence the dark and light isochromatic fringes, Figures 7.3 and 7.4. This interference is of course wavelength dependent so fringes are only clearly defined dark and light regions if a monochromatic light source is used. The resulting fringes are loci of constant principal stress difference, or constant shear stress, and are identified by number as they appear sequentially with increasing model loads. They may be related to actual stresses by the following simple formula:

$$\sigma_1 - \sigma_2 = \frac{Nf_\sigma}{t} \qquad\qquad (7.1)$$

where

$\sigma_{1,2}$ = principal stresses,
N = fringe order,
f_σ = material fringe value,
t = model thickness.

The separation of principal stress magnitudes is not easily performed, however fringes at a free boundary are directly related to the tangential principal stress since the normal stress is zero. The quarter wave plates illustrated in Figure 7.1 are used to permit viewing of isochromatic fringes without the isoclinic fringes being superimposed (Sharples, 1981).

7.2 PHOTOELASTICITY IN BIOMECHANICS

Photoelastic methods have been applied to biomechanical studies since the late 1930s, particularly to investigate stresses in bone and implants in the orthopaedic (Orr *et al.*, 1990) and dental fields. In orthopaedic engineering the first application of photoelastic methods was described by Milch (1940) with reference to stresses in the upper end of the femur. The ready indication of principal stress directions has made photoelastic methods particularly suitable for study of the directional properties of cancellous bone and its response to orthopaedic procedures (Fessler, 1957; Chand *et al.*, 1976; Steen-Jensen, 1978a; Pauwels, 1980). A particularly interesting analysis of the neck of the femur was reported by Williams and Svensson (1971). This work was unusual in deriving the distribution of stresses in the outer cortical bone and inner cancellous bone and hence taking the non-homogeneous nature of the bone into account. Orthopaedic implants present fewer problems in

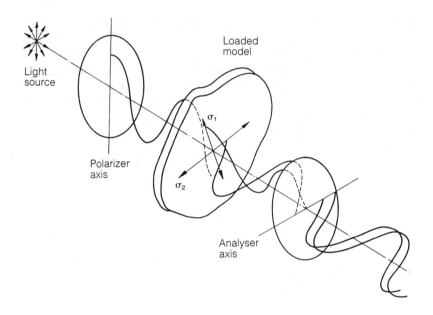

Figure 7.3 Interference of light causing isochromatic fringes.

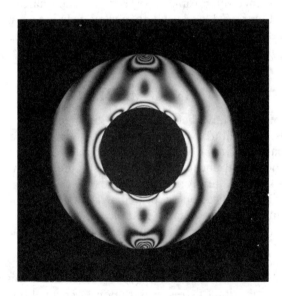

Figure 7.4 Isochromatic fringes in a ring loaded in compression on the vertical diameter.

photoelastic modelling due to their predictable material properties yet relatively few applications have been reported. An early study by Haboush (1952) had the aim of measuring stresses in implants for fixing femoral neck fractures at different attitudes of insertion. A similar study was subsequently performed by Steen-Jensen (1978b). The stress analysis of joint replacement components has not attracted many photoelastic investigations, however some experiments have been reported concerning stresses in the femoral stems of hip prostheses and in the surrounding cement mantle (Kennedy *et al.*, 1979; Orr *et al.*, 1985, 1986). Recent studies of the stresses in ceramic femoral heads, due to taper mounting on prosthetic stems, report applications of the frozen stress method (Fessler and Fricker, 1989; Andrisano *et al.*, 1990). Fixation of joint replacements is an important area of research to which photoelastic studies can make a useful contribution but necessarily involves the modelling of bone as well as implants and bone cement (Miles and McNamee, 1989).

The applications of photoelastic methods to model dental structures reflect developments in restorative dentistry since 1949. Early publications generally relate to cavity restorations in teeth (Noonan, 1949; Granath, 1964). Investigation of stresses in designs of removable partial dentures followed with later investigation of fixed bridges (El-Ebrashi *et al.*, 1970; Farah *et al.*, 1979).

Photoelastic techniques have been used during the last decade not only to study fixed and removable prostheses but to contribute to the development of dental implants where direct fixation of prostheses is made to the bones of the jaw (Atmaram and Mohammed, 1981).

The application of photoelastic methods to natural materials requires assumptions, the most common being the validity of representing three-dimensional structures by two-dimensional projections of their shape and the possible restrictions of representing the non-homogeneous, non-isotropic structure of bone by thermosetting plastic models. Such considerations are addressed by many authors and it has been demonstrated that they need not preclude successful investigations using photoelastic models (Fessler, 1957; Williams and Svennson, 1971; Holm, 1981).

7.3 PHOTOELASTIC METHODS

Photoelastic experiments may be conveniently classified as using two-dimensional or three-dimensional models. Two-dimensional experiments are desirable, if realistically able to represent the structure being studied, due to ease of manufacture and ready application and variation of loading. Biomechanical models tend to represent objects of irregular shape and the technique of milling models from sheet

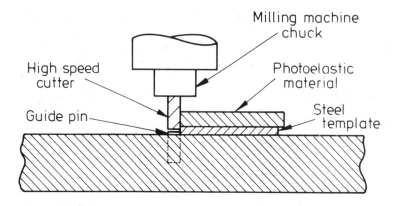

Figure 7.5 Machining two-dimensional model to a template.

material by hand, whilst being guided by a metal template, has been found to be very successful (Dally and Riley, 1965), Figure 7.5. Light cuts and sharp cutters prevent residual edge stresses (Fessler, 1974). Care should be taken that the model material is well bonded to the metal template to prevent relative movement during machining, noting however that the two components must be separated later without damage to the model. The availability of CNC milling facilities is useful if a model requires closely conforming parts without stress concentrations due to localized points of contact (Orr *et al.*, 1985).

Loading of two-dimensional models is usually not difficult but care should be taken to avoid buckling out of the model plane. Problems of this type may be solved by supporting models between sheets of optically insensitive material such as 'Perspex'. Levers and wires loaded by weights have been found to be most satisfactory means of loading since, unlike spring devices, load magnitudes do not vary with deformation of the model.

Three-dimensional modelling is usually performed using the 'Frozen Stress Technique' on which much advice is available (Dally and Riley, 1965; Fessler and Perla, 1973; Fessler, 1974, 1977). This technique relies on subjecting a thermosetting plastic model to loading while it undergoes a heating and cooling cycle. The cycle reaches the critical temperature for the plastic at which its elastic modulus markedly decreases allowing greater deformation than occurred when loading at room temperature. This deformation, which causes the double refraction properties, is maintained when loading is removed on cooling and the model may be sectioned to examine stresses in a series of two-dimensional slices.

The casting of models can cause problems due to residual stresses and air being trapped in moulds. The irregular shape of natural structures such as bones make the use of a flexible mould attractive since the embedded pattern or prototype can be extracted merely by slitting the mould material. Models can be cast in thermosetting silicone rubber moulds provided that they are small and the rubber does not deform due to its own weight. The low elastic modulus of the mould material accommodates changes in model dimensions due to contraction on cooling without imposing significant residual stresses. Larger moulds require more rigid materials to maintain their geometrical integrity but may be lined with silicone rubber to prevent the model being stressed due to differences in contraction between the model and mould. The entrapment of air can be overcome by careful venting and orientation of the mould. It has been found helpful to raise the recommended pouring temperature of 'Araldite CT200' by approximately 10°C to lower its viscosity and aid the escape of bubbles. It is also helpful to pour the liquid resin in contact with the runner wall to prevent air being carried into the mould.

7.4 SPECIFIC APPLICATIONS OF PHOTOELASTIC METHODS

7.4.1 Two-dimensional modelling of a hip prosthesis stem and bone cement

A two-dimensional model of a 'Charnley' hip prosthesis was made to investigate the effects of orientation on stresses in the femoral stem (Orr *et al.*, 1985). The stem and socket profiles were cut using a CNC milling machine in order to achieve a closely conforming fit between the parts. The material used was 'Araldite CT200' in sheet form, 6 mm thick. Loading was applied to the head of the two-dimensional model by a lever and weights, with a ball bearing mounted carriage between the lever and model to ensure that no horizontal components of force were applied as the model deformed. The resulting isochromatic fringe patterns were recorded by tracing on predrawn stem profiles. Edge stresses were plotted in terms of fringe orders, represented by the perpendicular distances from the plotted line to the stem boundaries, Figure 7.6. The maximum fringe orders on the medial and lateral stem surfaces were determined. The fringe orders are directly proportional to principal stress differences, however since there was negligible contact stress over most of the stem surfaces the fringe orders plotted are proportional to the bending stresses parallel to these free boundaries. Figure 7.7 shows the variation of boundary stresses, expressed as multiples of fringe order, with prosthesis orientation relative to the applied joint force.

A subsequent study was conducted using a stem of the same shape

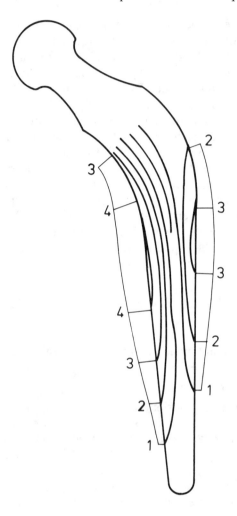

Figure 7.6 Boundary fringe orders for a two-dimensional model hip prosthesis.

as in the previous experiment to examine the effects of resorption of the proximal bone of the femur on cement stresses (Humphreys, 1990). The photoelastic part of the model, representing the cement layer, was made from CR39 or 'Columbia Resin' ($E = 2$ GPa) while the femoral stem was machined from aluminium ($E = 70$ GPa) and the surrounding bone socket from 'Tufnol' ($E = 5.5$ GPa), a fabric reinforced phenolic resin. A diagram of the assembled model is shown in Figure 7.8.

The model was loaded as in the previous experiment and fringes recorded in the cement layer, prior to reducing the support height of the medial wall of the socket in 5 mm increments. As before higher

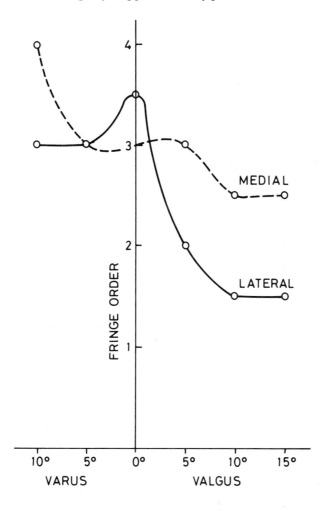

Figure 7.7 Maximum fringe orders with variation of medio-lateral orientation.

fringe orders were recorded in varus positions compared to valgus and maximum fringe orders increased markedly as loosening was simulated by removal of medial support, Figure 7.9. It was noted that tensile bending stresses were occurring in the medial cement layer during the experiments. The maximum tensile stresses measured during the experiments are presented in Figure 7.10, which demonstrates trends for cement stresses under compromised support. The photoelastic results were used to guide the positioning of electrical resistance strain gauges to measure the bending and hoop stresses in the cement and evaluate the likelihood of failure.

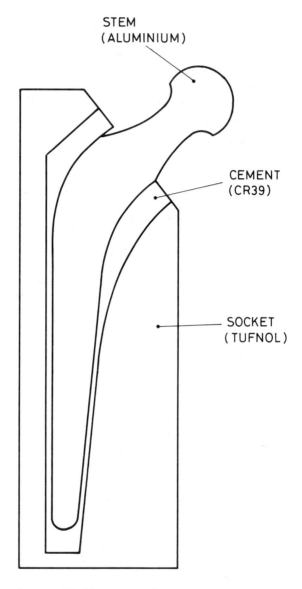

Figure 7.8 Photoelastic model of bone cement layer.

7.4.2 Three-dimensional modelling of the talus

A three-dimensional modelling approach was used to investigate the directions of principal stresses in the talus for comparison with the architecture of the internal cancellous bone. A talus was obtained from an anatomical specimen and embedded in silicone rubber casting

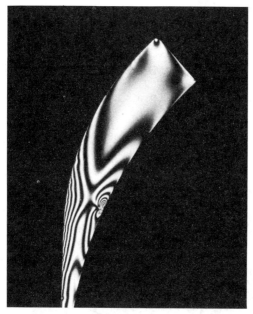

Figure 7.9 Isochromatic fringes in medial cement layer with reduced support.

material as described above. Impressions were also cast from the tibia and fibula and the socket in the foot for replication in plaster. These were later used to load the photoelastic models. The models of the talus were stress free, by observation in the polariscope, after casting and curing, again using 'Araldite CT200'.

A range of models were stress frozen at different positions of ankle flexion/extension. Each model was loaded by replica articular surfaces through a thin layer of the silicone rubber casting material to prevent stress concentrations due to incongruities of the contacting surfaces or due to differential contraction of model and loading materials during the cooling phase of the stress freezing cycle. The stress frozen models were successfully sectioned using a sharp bandsaw at low cutting speed whilst directing a jet of cold air over the cutting area to prevent heating of the model. The cut faces of the slices were smoothed by hand on wet abrasive paper on a flat, plate glass base. Paper was used down to approximately 600 grit size. If rubbing is continued for too long there is a tendency for edges to become rounded and hence boundary fringes distorted, since model thickness is a factor determining isochromatic fringe order at any point. The above grade of abrasive leaves a slightly opaque surface on the model but the transmission of light is greatly enhanced if a trace of glycerine is applied. The slices obtained were mounted in the polariscope and the isoclinic fringe loci recorded by tracing, for subsequent derivation of isostatic lines and comparison

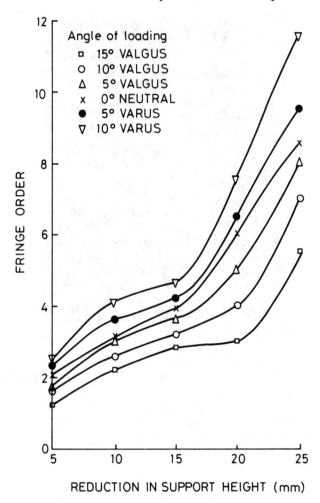

Figure 7.10 Maximum fringe orders due to tensile stresses in cement mantle.

with the structure of a corresponding slice from the actual bone. In a frozen stress model isochromatic fringes will generally also be visible so care should be taken to identify the isoclinic fringes correctly, especially avoiding confusion with the zero order isochromatic which is also black when viewed in white light. Of course the isochromatic fringes do not move as the polarizer and analyser are rotated. The isochromatic fringe patterns can be observed without confusion by using the quarter wave plates as described above, Figure 7.11. The orientation of the internal stress field was found to vary with ankle joint position and tended to match the cancellous bone structure at the push-off stage of stance.

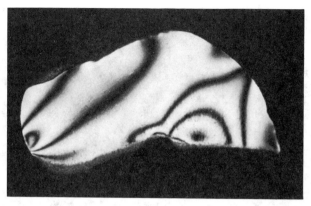

Figure 7.11 Isochromatic fringes in a slice from a frozen stress model of the talus.

7.4.3 Frozen stress modelling of dental bridges

A project to investigate stresses in dental bridges and their bonding to adjacent teeth was performed in association with the University Department of Restorative Dentisty. Preliminary frozen stress models of teeth demonstrated that analysis was difficult with life size models. This was due to inadequate fringe orders being visible in model sections which were rather thin (<1 mm). This problem was successfully overcome by casting models from a set of replicas of human teeth 2.5 times life size. The materials used for the teeth and bridge components were PLM–4 and PLM–9 photoelastic materials as supplied from Measurements Group Inc., PO Box 27777, Raleigh, NC, USA. These modern materials were chosen for their ratio of stiffnesses of 2.41, which is close to the ratio of 2.16 for the prototype materials of enamel and the metal bridge. The teeth were inserted in a base representing the jaw with an intervening layer of silicone rubber to permit relative movement of the teeth in their sockets. The bridge was prepared by a lost wax casting method in silicone rubber casting material. The bridge was bonded to the adjacent teeth using an adhesive normally used for photoelastic coatings. A series of these models was made, to be stress frozen under loading at different positions on the bridge and teeth. Models were made to represent posterior and anterior bridges.

Sections were carefully cut to allow examination of stresses in the body of the bridge itself and also in the supporting arms which were bonded to the teeth. Both isochromatic fringes and isoclinic fringes were recorded and isostatic lines derived. Stresses in the supporting arms were of particular interest, isochromatic fringes in a bridge design with perforated arms being shown in Figure 7.12. It was found that

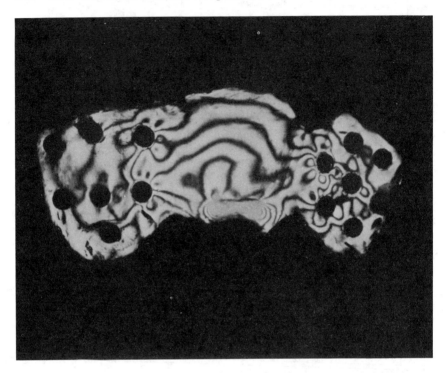

Figure 7.12 Isochromatic fringes in a dental bridge with perforated bonding arms.

while sectioning and inspection in a transmission polariscope was necessary for the body of the bridge, reflection methods were very suitable for examination of the supporting arms. The adhesive used was reflective and the arms were substantially of constant thickness (approximately 2 mm), so the conditions for viewing with a reflection polariscope were satisfied. The advantages were greater fringe orders being visible, for a given deformation, due to the double passage of light through the model and fringes could be observed while the model was subjected to a variety of direct loadings without the need for stress freezing or sectioning.

7.5 DEVELOPMENTS IN THE APPLICATION OF PHOTOELASTIC METHODS IN BIOMECHANICS

The number of papers published which describe photoelastic investigations of biomechanical structures appear to be increasing. In the orthopaedic and dental fields more papers have been published during the past decade than in any previously from the initial applications of photoelastic techniques. The use of photoelasticity is still not very common but awareness of the techniques is spreading. Two-dimensional experiments are by far the most convenient to conduct but the geometry of natural structures often needs a three-dimensional approach. Even with this type of modelling there will be many questions regarding the validity of models, for example concerning non-homogeneity, non-isotropy, assumptions about loading and boundary conditions. These must be addressed when planning experiments but need not prevent useful results being obtained within the limitations of the assumptions.

The frozen stress technique of three-dimensional modelling is well developed although casting and loading methods often require some innovation for particular applications. The sectioning of models requires decisions regarding which planes to view but now this may be accomplished non-destructively using scattered light photoelasticity (Kihara *et al.*, 1985, 1987). This concept is attractive but interpretation of results is not straightforward.

New applications for even simple two-dimensional experiments can easily be identified in the biomechanical field. There is plenty of scope for researchers to introduce photoelastic experiments into their work and develop expertise in the methods described. The main equipment required is commonly found in mechanical engineering departments and so it is often possible to start work or evaluate the methods with minimal expense. Photoelastic stress analysis is one of the longer established experimental techniques but it has not been supplanted by more recent experimental and theoretical methods, indeed it often proves valuable in complementing results from other sources.

REFERENCES

Andrisano, A.O., Dragoni, E. and Strozzi, A. (1990) Axisymmetric mechanical analysis of ceramic heads for total hip replacement. *Proc. I. Mech. E., Part H: Engng. Med.*, **204**, 157–67.

Atmaram, G.H. and Mohammed, H. (1981) Photoelastic stress analysis of dental implants with different root configurations. *N.Y. State Dent. J.*, **47**, 30–3.

Chand, R., Haug, E. and Rim, K. (1976) Stresses in the human knee joint. *J. Biomech.*, **9**, 417–22.

Dally, J.W. and Riley, W.F. (1965) *Experimental Stress Analysis*, McGraw-Hill, New York.

El-Ebrashi, M.K., Craig, R.G. and Peyton, F.A. (1970) Experimental stress analysis of dental restorations Part 7. Structural design and stress analysis of fixed partial dentures. *J. Prosthet. Dent.*, **23**, 177.

Farah, J.W., MacGregor, A.R. and Miller, T.P.G. (1979) Stress analysis of disjunct removable partial dentures. *J. Prosthet. Dent.*, **42**, 271–5.

Fessler, H. (1957) Load distribution in a model of a hip joint. *J. Bone Jt. Surg.*, **39**, 145–53.

Fessler, H. (1974) On the general problems of static experimental stress analysis, in *Quaderni de La Ricerca Scientifica, 85*, Consiglio Nazionale Delle Ricerche, Rome.

Fessler, H. (1977) *Applications of Photoelasticity*, Monograph on methods and practice for stress and strain measurement, British Society for Strain Measurement, Newcastle upon Tyne.

Fessler, H. and Fricker, D.C. (1989) A study of stresses in alumina universal heads of femoral prostheses. *Proc. I. Mech. E., Part H: Engng. Med.*, **203H**, 15–34.

Fessler, H. and Perla, M. (1973) Precision casting of epoxy-resin photoelastic models. *J. Strain Anal.*, **8**, 30–4.

Frocht, M.M. (1941) *Photoelasticity*, John Wiley, New York, p. 99.

Granath, L.E. (1964) Further photoelastic studies on the restorations between the cavity and occlusal portion of Class 2 restorations. *Odent. Rev.*, **15**, 290–8.

Haboush, E.J. (1952) Photoelastic stress and strain analysis in cervical fractures of the femur. *Bulletin Hosp. Jt. Dis.*, **13**, 252–8.

Holm, N.J. (1981) The development of a two dimensional stress-optical model of the os coxae. *Acta Orthop. Scand.*, **52**, 608–18.

Humphreys, P.K. (1990) An investigation into the fixation and endurance of hip replacements, PhD thesis, The Queen's University of Belfast, pp. 92–100.

Kennedy, F.E., Collier, J.P. and Komornik, L.A. (1979) An experimental study of the stress distribution in bone cement used to grout standard and porous coated hip prostheses. *Adv. Bioengng.*, ASME Annual Meeting, pp. 75–8.

Kihara, T., Unno, M., Kitada, C., Kubo, H. and Nagata, R. (1985) Three dimensional stress distribution measurement in a model of the human ankle joint by scattered-light polarizer photoelasticity, Part 1. *Appl. Opt.*, **24**, 3363–7.

Kihara, T., Unno, M., Kitada, C., Kubo, H. and Nagata, R. (1987) Three dimensional stress distribution measurement in a model of the human ankle joint by scattered-light polarizer photoelasticity: Part 2. *Appl. Opt.*, **26**, 643–9.

Kuske, A. and Robertson, G. (1974) *Photoelastic Stress Analysis*, John Wiley, London.

Milch, H. (1940) Photoelastic studies of bone forms. *J. Bone Jt. Surg.*, **22**, 621–6.

Miles, A.W. and McNamee, P.B. (1989) Strain gauge and photoelastic evaluation of the load transfer in the pelvis in total hip replacement: The effect of the position of the axis of rotation. *Proc. I. Mech. E., Part H: Engng. Med.*, **203H**, 103–7.

Noonan, M.A. (1949) The use of photoelasticity in the study of cavity preparations. *J. Dent. Child.*, **16**, 24–8.

Orr, J.F., James, W.V. and Bahrani, A.S. (1985) A preliminary study of the effects of medio-lateral rotation on stresses in an artificial hip joint. *Engng. Med.*, **14**, 39–42.

Orr, J.F., James, W.V. and Bahrani, A.S. (1986) The effects of hip prosthesis stem cross-sectional profile on the stresses induced in bone cement. *Engng. Med.*, **15**, 13–18.

Orr, J.F., Humphreys, P.K., James, W.V. and Bahrani, A.S. (1990) The application of photoelastic techniques in orthopaedic engineering, in *Applied Stress Analysis* (eds T.H. Hyde and E. Ollerton), Elsevier Applied Science, Barking.

Pauwels, F. (1980) *Biomechanics of the Locomotor Apparatus*, Springer-Verlag, Berlin.

Sharples, K. (1981) Photoelastic stress analysis. *Chartered Mech. Eng.*, **28** (9), 42–50

Steen-Jenson, J. (1978a) A photoelastic study of the proximal femur. *Acta Orthop. Scand.*, **49**, 54–9.

Steen-Jenson, J. (1978b) A photoelastic study of the hip nail-plate in unstable trochanteric fractures. *Acta Orthop. Scand.*, **49**, 60–4.

Williams, J.F. and Svensson, N.L. (1971) An experimental stress analysis of the neck of the femur. *Med. Biol. Engng.*, **9**, 479–93.

8

Photoelastic coating techniques

J.B. Finlay

8.1 INTRODUCTION

Strain measurements in orthopaedic biomechancis often involve bone with its characteristic anisotropic mechanical properties. Photoelastic coatings offer one mechanism for monitoring the full-field distribution of shear strains on the bone. These coatings are ideally suited for monitoring areas involving strain concentrations. The technique, however, involves certain limitations such as reinforcement of the test-piece. The strengths and limitations of the technique are discussed in terms of references in both the engineering and orthopaedic literature.

Conventional transmission-photoelasticity has the advantage of providing a full-field picture of the shear-strains within a two-dimensional or three-dimensional model of a structure or device. For orthopaedic applications, transmission-photoelasticity has the disadvantage that the complex anisotropic structural organization of the soft and hard connective tissues are represented in the model by an homogeneous isotropic plastic. A possible technique for overcoming these problems was described by Mesnager (1930). He proposed the use of a birefringent material attached by a reflective coating to the surface of a structure of interest; however, his available coating was glass which provided significant problems of reinforcement and contouring. Subsequently, Oppel (1937) described the use of Bakelite as a coating material. The unavailability of adequate adhesives and its limitation to flat surfaces restricted the application of this technique. In the 1950s, developments in France (Fleury and Zandman, 1954), the United States (D'Agostino et al., 1955a, b) and Japan (Kawata, 1958) led to the development of the technology for the successful industrial application of reflective photoelastic coatings. The background of the development and the theory for the application of photoelastic coatings are well described in the monograph by Zandman et al. (1977a).

The theory for reflective photoelastic coatings is similar to that applied to transmission-photoelasticity which has been dealt with briefly in Chapter 7. The strain-optic law relates the principal strains (ϵ_1 and ϵ_2) to the number of fringes (N), the wavelength of light (λ), the thickness of the sample (t) and the sensitivity-constant (k) for the plastic material, by the relationship:

$$\epsilon_1 - \epsilon_2 = N\lambda/(2kt) \tag{8.1}$$

The 2 in the denominator of the equation identifies the difference between photoelastic coatings and transmission-photoelasticity, in that the photoelastic coating requires the polarized light to pass through the coating before being reflected (by an aluminium-impregnated cement) back through the plastic to be viewed by the analyser. The plastic coating is initially cast as a flat sheet of about 2 mm thickness and, while it is in a pliable phase of curing, it is moulded to the surface of the structure of interest. Subsequently, during a 16 h period, the plastic hardens to take the shape of the structure under study. After the plastic has hardened, it can be cleaned and attached to the structure (e.g. bone) with a reflective cement which again requires 12 h or more to harden.

The quantitative assessment of photoelastic data requires an understanding of isochromatics (lines connecting points of equal magnitude of shear strain) and isoclinics (lines connecting points whose principal direct strains have the same direction). These techniques are well described by Zandman *et al.* (1977b).

8.2 REVIEW OF RELEVANT TECHNIQUES

In the use of photoelastic coatings, it must be remembered that the isochromatic fringes represent the shear strain in the system, i.e. the difference between the principal direct strains. Therefore, a structure under uniform tension (such as a pressure vessel) will experience principal direct strains that are equal. Consequently, in such a case, the shear strain will be zero and the photoelastic coating will provide no signal. This feature needs to be taken into account, when selecting photoelastic coatings as a potential strain transducer.

Since the photoelastic coatings indicate the magnitude of the shear strains on the surface of a structure, they are most readily applied to the analysis of structures whose failure criterion is best described by shear strain. Such is the case with brittle materials which can characterize the behaviour of old bone, but not new bone. The failure of ductile materials seems to be well represented by the Von Mises failure criterion (Johnson, 1987; Raghava *et al.*, 1973). More complex failure criteria have been suggested for the analysis of orthopaedic materials such as polymethylmethacrylate bone cement, where a strain-energy density criterion has been proposed (Vasu *et al.*, 1983).

The foregoing section indicates a necessity for computing direct strains and, in particular, principal direct strains from the photoelastic data. O'Regan (1965) and Zandman *et al.* (1977c) indicated that the use of strips of photoelastic coating could be used for computing direct strains. The thin strip of coating is relatively insensitive to transverse strains and, consequently, the photoelastic signal basically derives from the longitudinal strain in the plastic strip. The use of three strips, applied at different times and different angles, to a spot on the surface of a specimen will yield three direct strains which will permit computation of the principal strains, i.e. as with the application of strain-gauge rosettes.

Another approach to the derivation of the direct strains is to obtain another photoelastic reading but with the light passing along a different path through the coating. An 'oblique incidence attachment' is used on the polariscope to provide this path (Redner, 1963). This technique and the associated theory is well described by Zandman *et al.* (1977d). The oblique incidence attachment, however, is cumbersome and difficult to apply, especially on curved surfaces. In an attempt to solve this problem, a commercially-available 'stress separator gauge' has been developed (Measurements Group, 1986). The gauge involves two elements at 90° to one another, so that the sum of their strains will be constant, regardless of the orientation of the gauge (a feature which is readily appreciated by reference to the Mohr's strain circle). The photoelastic coating provides a signal which is proportional to the difference of the two principal strains, while the separator gauge is used to compute a signal which is equal to the sum of the two direct strains; consequently, the individual direct strains may be computed from the two simultaneous equations. Strain gauges, however, will create reinforcement of low modulus materials (Perry, 1984). The separator gauge relies on a construction that minimizes local reinforcement effects when installed on photoelastic plastic. Furthermore, the reinforcement error is claimed to be entirely eliminated by calibrating the gauge for its 'effective' gauge factor when installed on standard coatings (Measurements Group, 1986). If coatings of the same thickness are always applied to structures with the same modulus of elasticity, and the combinations of tension and bending are the same in each test, then such claims may be appropriate; however, researchers should make attempts to verify these assumptions before applying such calculations to their experimental data.

8.3 APPLICATIONS IN ORTHOPAEDICS

While the text by Zandman *et al.* (1977e) refers to applications of photoelastic coatings to the skull, the femur and the human jaw, there are no references to these various reports. Frankel and Burstein (1970) showed an example of a photoelastic coating on a loaded femur with two drill-holes in it; however, their text provided no discussion of the technique or the results. The most complete report, utilizing photoelastic coatings in an orthopaedic application, was by DiNovo (1985) who reported the use of the material on a fibre-composite model of bone fitted with a fracture-fixation plate. DiNovo, however, did not mention the thickness of the photoelastic coating used on the bone model which had an outer diameter of 25.4 mm and an inner diameter of 19 mm. The report also failed to address the potential reinforcement errors introduced by this coating. Curiously, the published figures by DiNovo, for the non-plated bone-model loaded in four-point bending, showed a shift in the neutral axis (i.e. the zero-order isochromatic) as the bending-moment increased from 31.2 N m through 54.6 to 73.3 N m. This feature was not described in the manuscript and possibly relates to a certain amount of artistic licence (!) in the hand-drawn figures illustrating the fringe orders.

In applications to orthopaedic problems, the absence of comprehensive manuscripts evaluating its qualitative and, particularly, its quantitative potentials clearly represents a problem for future routine applications of photoelastic coatings. In a brief abstract, Jones and Hungerford (1987) attempted to validate the use of photoelastic coatings on human femora by comparing the data with strain-gauge information. On the basis of obtaining a linear relationship between the shear strains monitored by the strain gauge and those monitored by the photoelastic coating (shear strain monitored by the strain gauge equalled 1.5 times the shear strain monitored by the photoelastic coating), they concluded that the photoelastic coatings provided an accurate quantitative technique.

Based on the various reports in the literature, it would appear that photoelastic coatings should not necessarily be employed as a precise quantitative system for assessing stresses or strains. The technique, however, provides an excellent full-field presentation of the general distribution of strains and, thereby, permits the identification of severely under-strained or over-strained areas. In such extreme conditions, the precise magnitude of the problem is of little relevance in a practical problem. The solution to the problem is to add material, remove material, modify the shape, etc., and then to re-evaluate the structure with a photoelastic coating, possibly prior to the application of strain gauges or some other transducer technique to obtain more precise quantitative information if it is required.

Hungerford and his co-workers (Jones and Hungerford, 1987; Wuh *et al.*, 1986), as well as Walker and his colleagues (Walker and Robertson, 1988; Zhou *et al.*, 1988), have used the technique in studying the changes in femoral strains associated with hip implants, while Finlay *et al.* (1986, 1989) have reported the use of photoelastic coatings as preliminary full-field strain analyses before subsequent detailed strain-gauge investigations of total hip replacements in the pelvis and femur, respectively.

The display of contours of constant shear strain (isochromatics) reveals a certain amount of information about the strains within a structure; however, information on the principal direct strains may be of equal or greater significance. Consequently, the newcomer to stress analysis may wish to have data on the principal shear strains, the principal direct strains, and the trajectories of the principal direct strains (isostatics). As with many analytical techniques, the experienced analyst can readily focus on areas of concern, without resort to tedious plotting processes. The explanation of the results, however, to a lay audience may well require the plotting of such information – especially isostatics. Blum (1977) has noted that '. . . plotting the stress trajectories is laborious and generally not essential to finding a solution to a given problem. However, it can bring things into focus, and greatly enhance the understanding of the behaviour of a structure under load. . .'.

Kummer (1966) used a photoelastic model to study the isostatics in the femoral head and proximal regions of a model femur with an abductor-muscle simulation. A grid of dots was oriented with the polarizing lens and the grid was superimposed upon isoclinic fringes recorded at 10° intervals. Subsequently, each dotted isoclinic was printed on top of each other and the resulting pattern provided a good representation of the isostatics within the model. Subsequently, Holm (1981) applied this technique, with elaborate descriptions, to an analysis of the isostatics on a human pelvis around the acetabulum.

The use of quarter wave plates permits isoclinics to be removed from isochromatics when recording photoelastic data (Zandman *et al.*, 1977b). There is, however, no way of obtaining isoclinic information that is completely devoid of isochromatic data. The techniques described by Holm (1981) and Kummer (1966) rely on the absence of isochromatic fringes in the recording of isoclinic data. To some extent, this objective is obtained by applying a very small load so that there is no development of a first-order fringe. For many models, however, the isoclinic data will still include erronous dark areas which are not isoclinics but are, in fact, the zero-order isochromatics. The zero-order isochromatics will not move as the polarizing lens is rotated; however, they are not easily removed by conventional photographic techniques.

8.4 TIPS ON APPLICATION/INTERPRETATION

8.4.1 Materials and casting

In general, the techniques of application and analysis of photoelastic coatings are well described in the text by Zandman *et al.* (1977a) and in the various technical notes provided by the manufacturer of these materials. Some commonly encountered problems, however, are worth mentioning.

The solutions used for casting the photoelastic plastic have a high water content; consequently, once a tin has been opened it is susceptible to dehydration. Depending upon the extent of dehydration, the polymerization times may well vary from one batch of cast plastic to another batch. It is not advisable, therefore, to purchase large tins of the liquid plastic, unless it is anticipated that the open tin will be used within a few weeks.

A typical sheet of 200 mm × 200 mm × 2 mm thick will require 13.7 g of hardener with 76.6 g of resin. The viscosity of these liquids is such that a certain amount of the material clings to the side of any measuring vessel. Consequently, attempts to make very small sheets, of the order of 100 mm × 100 mm, can be frustrated by inaccuracies in the quantities of hardener and resin that are mixed together. These inaccuracies lead to quite unpredictable polymerization times. Many orthopaedic applications lend themselves to the routine use of 200 mm × 200 mm sheets.

A further aid in obtaining consistent results during polymerization is the use of a temperature-controlled plate. This device is now a standard piece of equipment supplied by the manufacturer of these plastics.

PL–1 liquid casting-plastic (Measurements Group, 1983) has been the most commonly used material in orthopaedic applications of photo-elastic coatings. While it is 25% more sensitive to shear strain than PL–8 plastic, after casting it discolours in a matter of weeks. PL–8, however, remains crystal clear and usable for years after it has been cast. This feature of discoloration is generally not described in the technical bulletins or scientific literature. Consequently, for many applications in education and research, PL–8 is the more appropriate choice.

8.4.2 Photography

The illumination provided by the reflection polariscope is rather limited and, consequently, a test sample may be shrouded in darkness and so provide a non-photogenic picture. This problem may be overcome by hanging a drape at some distance behind the test sample and illuminating it with another lamp. In this way, the edge of the test sample may be clearly defined.

Since the standard reflection polariscope employs a tungsten lamp, appropriate photographic film and/or filters need to be employed, in order to obtain the true colours of the isochromatics. Since the use of filters on a camera lens generally involves some loss of light and a requirement for a greater aperture (with its associated lower depth-of-focus), it is easier to bypass the use of filters by using colour film that is balanced for tungsten light, e.g. Kodak Ektachrome balanced for tungsten light (EPY). The choice of film-speed is optional; however, the 64 ASA film gives good resolution.

A static recording of isochromatic fringes does not necessarily give a feeling for the magnitude of the strains, unless there is a well-defined strain concentration within the picture. Loading a sample quasi-statically (i.e. at a low strain rate) or dynamically (at a higher strain rate), either with a triangular or sinusoidal wave form, gives an immediate impression of the areas where the strains are changing most rapidly as the load changes. Consequently, video-recording of dynamically-applied or quasi-statically-applied load helps in the visualization of differences in strain magnitude across the coated surface.

Many of the problems involved in the computation of isostatics by the techniques described by Kummer (1966) and Holm (1981) may be overcome using video-imaging and associated image-manipulation software. Using such equipment, isochromatic fringes, especially zero-order fringes, may be readily removed from the isoclinic data. The subsequent 'addition' of isoclinic data is then readily performed with such computer manipulation.

8.4.3 Potential errors

The major disadvantage of photoelastic coatings arises from two factors: the thickness of the coating, and the reinforcement the coating provides to the specimen. The coloured fringes, viewed in the coating, are a result of the strain distribution throughout the thickness of the coating; consequently, if there is a strain gradient from the surface of the specimen to the surface of the coating (due to bending effects, etc.), then the photoelastic effect will not be a true reflection of the strains at the surface of the specimen, Figure 8.1.

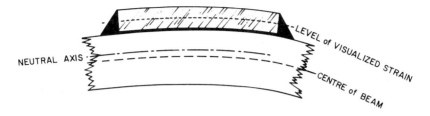

Figure 8.1 Depending upon the modulus of the substrate, the photoelastic coating may produce a reinforcement which will shift the neutral axis of bending. Also the 'effective' level of strain is at the centre of the coating, not at the surface of the specimen.

The most suitable commercial coating for use on bone has a modulus of elasticity of approximately 3 GPa. This latter modulus is comparable to the 10–20 GPa modulus of mid-diaphyseal cortical bone and, consequently, provides some localized reinforcement to the bone that it is monitoring. Since bones are rarely symmetrical in their cross-sectional shape, it cannot be assumed that a uniform coating around the bone will have no influence upon the location of the neutral axis of the bone. The reinforcement, apart from reducing the surface strains, also has the effect of moving the neutral axis of the specimen when it is subjected to bending loads. With simple beams, correction factors may be applied to take account of the reinforcement effects and movement of the neutral axis (Zandman *et al.*, 1977f); however, on complex structures such as bone, these correction factors do not represent a practical procedure, since the material properties of the bone (modulus of elasticity and Poisson's ratio) and the thickness of the cancellous and cortical bone are not known.

8.5 EXAMPLES IN ORTHOPAEDICS

As noted previously, detailed manuscripts of the application of photoelastic coatings to orthopaedic applications are rare (DiNovo, 1985; Walker and Robertson, 1988), with a number of other brief mentions of its use for qualitative illustrative purposes or the subsequent location of strain gauges (Frankel and Burstein, 1970; Zandman *et al.*, 1977e; Finlay *et al.*, 1986, 1989; Walker and Robertson, 1988).

As noted previously, a well-designed structure will show little isochromatic variation; however, orthopaedic procedures that require the drilling of holes in a bone may lead to interesting data from photoelastic coatings (Frankel and Burstein, 1970; Finlay *et al.*, 1985). A typical set of data are shown in Figure 8.2, around the pins supporting a fractured bone via an externally-applied fracture-fixation frame (Finlay *et al.*, 1985). In such applications, it is important that the photoelastic coating be cut back from the pin, so that the pin does not press on the coating during any deformation caused by the loading.

An interesting application of photoelastic coatings to the study of orthopaedic procedures on the human elbow is shown in Figure 8.3. In some individuals, a pathological bony growth develops around the olecranon fossa of the humerus (upper arm) as a result of impingement with the olecranon of the ulna (one of the bones of the forearm). The olecranon fossa is the depression seen in the ulna on the left of Figure 8.3. In the normal humerus, the bone within the olecranon fossa is very thin and appears translucent when held to the light. Since no major blood vessels pass through this bony membrane, any pathological bony growth may, therefore, be drilled out. This assumption has led to the development of a routine surgical procedure; however, surgeons were interested in validating this assumption and the full-field strain-monitoring capabilities of photoelastic coatings led to their use in this particular example. The coated samples were subjected separately to torsional and bending loads, both before and after the drilling of a hole. As expected, relatively uninteresting isochromatic data were obtained (i.e. strains represented by a single isochromatic colour), both before and after drilling the hole – except in the areas where the loads were applied. To remove these artefacts, the photo-elastic coating was removed in the regions of application of the load.

There is, perhaps, one fallacy in the assumptions related to this study of the elbow, in that normal bones were used for the study, i.e. due to the lack of availability of bones with the relatively unusual bony growths in the olecranon fossa. If the bony growths were allowed to develop for some time, then it is possible that the normal bone, reinforced by the bony growths, would remodel itself to involve a weaker central structure. Such remodelling takes place in the same way that muscles become smaller if they are not exercised. Drilling a hole in the 'remodelled' structure may, therefore, involve some more notable changes in the isochromatic strain patterns. Such information still needs to be elicited.

8.6 FUTURE DEVELOPMENTS

In their classic monograph on photoelastic coatings, Zandman *et al.* (1977g) described several potentially useful new developments for the technique of photoelastic coatings. The potential developments are still relevant and include: newer low-modulus, high-sensitivity plastics; the development of plastics that are more moisture-resistant and less susceptible to the aging effects that accompany current plastics; the development of more sensitive instruments for the measurement of low fringe-orders; and the potential use of holographic interferometry

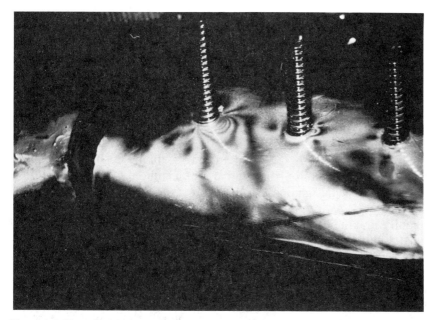

Figure 8.2 Photoelastic coatings are most impressive where stress concentrations exist. A typical example is shown at the pin–bone interface of an externally-applied fracture-fixation frame.

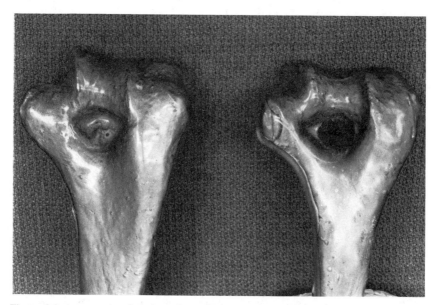

Figure 8.3 A new procedure in orthopaedic surgery of the elbow involves the removal (drilling out) of pathological bony growths in the olecranon fossa of the humerus. The photoelastically-coated bones, before and after drilling, are shown; however, the procedure appears to be benign and produces no notable fringes with either bending or torsional loads.

for the measurement of load-induced changes in thickness of the coating (a variation which is dependent upon the sum of the applied strains in the plane of the plastic). While the latter technique provides a non-contracting method for the determination of the principal direct strains, the subsequent development of the PhotoStress Separator Gauge (Measurements Group, 1986) has provided a more cost-effective approach to such calculations.

Personal computers have made a dramatic impact upon data analysis in engineering work. Software is readily available for using such computers in video analyses. While frame-grabbing techniques, image enhancement, and false-colouring are all techniques that would permit an impressive automation of the computation of isostatic data from isoclinic information, the processes are still somewhat tedious. Consequently, the major value of photoelastic coatings still appears to be in its full-field 'qualitative' visual presentation of information on shear strains. Acknowledging the limitations caused by reinforcement, etc., any quantitative data obtained from photoelastic coatings should be handled with care but may be seen as an additional advantage of the technique.

Photoelastic techniques, with all of their limitations and compromises, still offer a valuable full-field technique of strain analysis that can be employed in preliminary studies that are necessary to determine areas of concern in a practical structure. Subsequently, and if necessary, other non-contacting full-field techniques, strain-gauge analysis, and/or finite element analyses may be used more profitably than they could have been without the prior photoelastic analyses.

REFERENCES

Blum, A.E. (1977) The use and understanding of photoelastic coatings. *Strain*, **13**, 96–101.

D'Agostino, J., Drucker, D.C., Liu, C.K. and Mylonas, C. (1955a) An analysis of plastic behavior of metals with bonded birefringent plastics. *Proc. Soc. Exp. Stress Analysis*, **XII** (2), 115–22.

D'Agostino, J., Drucker, D.C., Liu, C.K. and Mylonas, C. (1955b) Epoxy adhesives and casting resins as photoelastic plastics. *Proc. Soc. Exp. Stress Analysis*, **XII** (2), 123–8.

DiNovo, J.A. (1985) A photoelastic coating technique for studying surface stress in bone plates. *J. Clin. Engng.*, **10** (2), 149–56.

Finlay, J.B., Bourne, R.B., Landsberg, R.P.D. and Andreae, P. (1986) Pelvic stresses *in vitro* – I. Malsizing of endoprostheses. *J. Biomech.*, **19**, 703–14.

Finlay, J.B., Rorabeck, C.H., Bourne, R.B., Armstrong, D. and Andreae, P.R. (1985) Pin-bone stresses associated with external fracture fixation. *Proc. 11th Can. Med. Biolog. Engng. Conf.*, pp. 89–90.

Finlay, J.B., Rorabeck, C.H., Bourne, R.B. and Tew, W.M. (1989) *In vitro* analysis of proximal femoral strains using PCA femoral implants and a hip-abductor muscle simulator. *J. Arthroplasty*, **4** (4), 335–45.

Fleury, R. and Zandman, F. (1954) Élasticité: Jauge d'efforts photoélastique. *Compt. Rendu.*, **238**, 1559–61.

Frankel, V.H. and Burstein, A.H. (1970) Elasticity, in *Orthopaedic Biomechanics. The Applications of Engineering to the Musculoskeletal System.* Lea & Febiger, Philadelphia, PA, pp. 40–76.

Holm, N. J. (1981) The development of a two-dimensional stress-optical model of the os coxae. *Acta Orthop. Scand.*, **52**, 135–43.

Johnson, R.P. (1987) Aids to effective design – FEM or BEM? *Chartered Mech. Engnr.*, **34** (9), 27–31.

Jones, L.C. and Hungerford, D.S. (1987) The photoelastic coating technique – its validation and use. *Trans. Orthop. Res. Soc.*, **12**, 406.

Kawata, K (1958) An analysis of elastoplastic behavior of metals by means of the photoelastic coating method. *J. Sci. Res. Inst. (Tokyo)*, **52**, 17–40.

Kummer, B. (1966) Photoelastic studies on the functional structure of bone. *Folia Biotheor.*, **6**, 31–40.

Measurements Group (1983) *Bulletin S–116–E. Materials for photoelastic coatings: Photostress ® method.* Measurements Group Inc., Raleigh, NC, pp. 1–7.

Measurements Group (1986) *Tech Note TN-708. Principal stress separation in Photostress ® measurements.* Measurements Group Inc., Raleigh, NC, pp. 1–8.

Mesnager, M. (1930) Sur la détermination optique des tensions intérieures dans les solides à trois dimensions. *Compt. Rendu.*, **190** (22), 1249–50.

Oppel, G. (1937) Das polarisationoptische Schichtverfahren zur Messung der Oberflächenspannungen am beanspruchten Bauteil ohne Modell. *Zeitschrift des Vereines Deutscher Ingenieure*, **81** (27), 803–4.

O'Regan, R. (1965) New method for determining strain on the surface of a body with photoelastic coatings. *Exptl. Mech.*, **5** (8), 241–6.

Perry, C.C. (1984) The resistance strain gauge revisited. *Exptl. Mech.*, **24** (4), 286–99.

Raghava, R., Caddell, R.M. and Yeh, G.S. (1973) The macroscopic yield behavior of polymers. *J. Mater. Sci.*, **8**, 225–32.

Redner, S.S. (1963) New oblique-incidence method for direct photoelastic measurement of principal strains. *Exptl. Mech.*, **3**, 67–72.

Vasu, R., Carter, D.R. and Harris, W.H. (1983) Evaluation of bone cement failure criteria with applications to the acetabular region. *J. Biomech. Engng.*, **105**, 332–7.

Walker, P.S. and Robertson, D.D. (1988) Design and fabrication of cementless hip stems. *Clin. Orthop.*, **235**, 25–34.

Wuh, H.C.K., Jones, L.C. and Hungerford, D.S. (1986) The effect of cementless femoral arthroplasty on stress transfer in the proximal femur. *Trans. Orthop. Res. Soc.*, **11**, 337.

Zandman, F., Redner, S. and Dally, J.W. (1977a) in *Photoelastic Coatings: SESA Monograph No. 3* (ed. B.E. Rossi), Society for Experimental Stress Analysis, Westport, CT, pp. 1–173.

Zandman, F., Redner, S. and Dally, J.W. (1977b) Properties of light and elementary theory of photoelasticity, in *Photoelastic Coatings: SESA Monograph No.*

3 (ed. B.E. Rossi), Society for Experimental Stress Analysis, Westport, CT, pp. 3–30.

Zandman, F., Redner, S. and Dally, J.W. (1977c) Elementary theory of photoelastic coatings, in *Photoelastic Coatings: SESA Monograph No. 3* (ed. B.E. Rossi), Society for Experimental Stress Analysis, Westport, CT, pp. 31–52.

Zandman, F., Redner, S. and Dally, J.W. (1977d) Instruments, in *Photoelastic Coatings: SESA Monograph No. 3* (ed. B.E. Rossi), Society for Experimental Stress Analysis, Westport, CT, pp. 66–84.

Zandman, F., Redner, S. and Dally, J.W. (1977e) Industrial and research applications, in *Photoelastic Coatings: SESA Monograph No. 3* (ed. B.E. Rossi), Society for Experimental Stress Analysis, Westport, CT, pp. 111–60.

Zandman, F., Redner, S. and Dally, J.W. (1977f) Parameters influencing analysis of data, in *Photoelastic Coatings: SESA Monograph No. 3* (ed. B.E. Rossi), Society for Experimental Stress Analysis, Westport, CT, pp. 85–110.

Zandman, F., Redner, S. and Dally, J.W. (1977g) Future developments, in *Photoelastic Coatings: SESA Monograph No. 3* (ed. B.E. Rossi), Society for Experimental Stress Analysis, Westport, CT, pp. 161–66.

Zhou, X-M., Robertson, D.D. and Walker, P.S. (1988) Femoral strain patterns with press-fit THR: A photoelastic analysis. *Trans. Orthop. Res. Soc.*, **13**, 350.

9
Holographic interferometry
J.C. Shelton

9.1 INTRODUCTION

The complex nature of bone structure constitutes one of the major problems in the investigation of mechanical systems in orthopaedics. Not only does the macroscopic architecture of the bones have to be considered, with the external and internal shapes of the bones differing from bone to bone, but also the complex anisotropy of cortical bone makes the mechanical properties difficult to model. In research into the fundamental aspects of orthopaedic practice, it is the analysis of the deformation which is of interest, whether it is of the bone itself, of an implant or of a composite system of a bone with an implant. If the loading conditions of the bone are massively disturbed then the bone will remodel to adjust to the new conditions and this frequently leads to a reduction in the stability of the implant–bone system as a result of extensive bone resorption. It is common for surgeons to attach overdesigned implants into the body, creating a large distortion in the loading patterns on the bone. Problems may occur in the months and years following implantation as the bone adapts its structure accordingly.

9.2 HOLOGRAPHY

Holography allows the reproduction of a wavefront of light, scattered by a three-dimensional object, by recording the intensity and phase of coherent monochromatic light which is reflected from the object. A record of this object wave, as compared to a reference beam, is made on a photographic emulsion, coated on a glass plate for physical stability. An ordinary photograph records only the intensity of the light reflected from an object producing a two-dimensional image. By recording the additional information of the phase of the wave it is

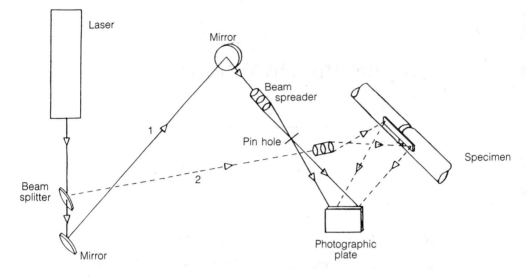

Figure 9.1 Experimental system for recording holograms.

possible to reconstruct completely an image of the object and view it in three dimensions. The theoretical basis of holography was first described by Gabor in 1948, but problems arose in the practical application of the theory, as an adequate monochromatic and coherent light source was not available (Erf, 1974). However with the development of the laser these difficulties were overcome.

The beam from a laser, producing both monochromatic and temporally coherent light, i.e. light of a constant wavelength and made up of waves which are the same over a period of time, is split into two parts known as a reference beam and an object beam, as shown in Figure 9.1. The reference beam is directed via a series of mirrors, through a diffuser and onto the photographic plate. The object beam is directed along a pathway of identical length, through a diffuser, and onto the object; this beam is scattered and some of the reflected light falls onto the photographic plate. The photographic plate is thus exposed to the reference and object beams simultaneously and the interference between the beams appears as a diffraction pattern which constitutes a hologram.

The reconstructed image can be viewed by replacing the processed photographic plate (or hologram) in its original position, and illuminating it using the reference beam *only*. The virtual* image of the object in three dimensions identical to the original object can then be seen by looking through the plate. It is possible to record either the virtual

* Virtual image – image generated in front of plate due to divergence of beams.

or the real† image photographically, but the information on the phase of the light is then lost.

9.3 INTERFEROMETRIC TECHNIQUES

Holographic interferometry can provide a detailed description of the surface displacements, although one hologram only gives a limited amount of information about the absolute displacements. The literature has many descriptions of holographic interferometry (Vest, 1979; Abramson, 1981; Jones and Wykes, 1983), however a brief summary of the techniques commonly used in biomechanics is included in the following sections.

9.3.1 Real time

If the superposition of light from the reference and object beams is viewed through a hologram of the same object, interference between two wavefronts can occur, provided that the processed holographic plate has been replaced exactly in its original position (to the nearest quarter wavelength of light) and the photographic emulsion has suffered minimal shrinkage during the development process. When the object is then displaced or deformed slightly interference causes alternate dark and light fringes to appear just in front of the object. This is a result of the change in the phase of the real object wavefront relative to that recorded on the plate. This technique produces a 'real-time' or 'live' holographic interference pattern (Vest, 1979). The fringe pattern depends on the type of deformation and the direction of viewing.

9.3.2 Double exposure

An alternative technique, which eliminates the problem of precise repositioning of the hologram, is known as the 'frozen fringe' or 'double exposure' hologram. The plate is never disturbed during the recording phase of this method, so that in practice it is easier to use than the real-time method. A hologram of an object is recorded in its undeformed state, the object is then deformed or undergoes a small displacement, and a second exposure is recorded on the same photographic plate. When processed the hologram reconstructs both images which interfere with each other so that interference fringes are superimposed on the image of the object. A single hologram records one loading condition and can be viewed in the absence of the object.

---

† Real image – image generated behind holographic plate.

Properly interpreted, a hologram can be used for strain and therefore stress analysis and the technique is commonly used for non-destructive testing.

There are several advantages of using holography rather than other more conventional techniques. Investigations by holography produce a high resolution, non-contacting image of the actual body; the deformation that is recorded is purely as a result of the loads that are applied to the object and is not, therefore, affected by the recording method. In addition the information relates to the actual object itself and it is not necessary to model the materials or structures. The technique records the deformations of an object, in and out of plane, which are approximately parallel to the line of sight and of the order of 0.5 μm. The sensitivity of the method depends on the geometrical arrangement that is used (Piwernetz, 1979), and also the wavelength of the laser light used. In the most general form it can be assumed that fringes occur as a result of out-of-plane displacements of $\lambda/2$ where λ is the wavelength of the light emitted from the laser. The technique of holography provides a two-dimensional display of the deformation of the surface of the object, which appears as interference fringes in front of its image. Broadly interpreted, these fringes provide an indication of the areas which have undergone a high strain, shown by a high fringe density, and this can be clearly seen without any further calculations.

However there are some disadvantages arising from the use of this technique. One of the major problems is the high sensitivity of the method, which means that only small deformations can be recorded, unless some desensitizing techniques, such as the elimination of rigid body motion, are used (Abramson, 1974). It is primarily the out-of-plane displacements that are recorded, as will be described in the following sections. However the technique also records fringes caused by rigid body motion, and in-plane deformation. These can be overcome by using sandwich holography (Saxby, 1989) but this increases the complexity of the system considerably.

9.4 INTERPRETATION OF DOUBLE EXPOSURE HOLOGRAPHY

The fringe pattern depends on all the individual components of the displacement present, i.e. the deformation, rotation and rigid body translations of the object. Two of the simplest methods for interpretation of the fringes, relating displacement or deformation to the fringes, are the zero fringe method and the fringe counting method (Briers, 1976; Vest, 1979).

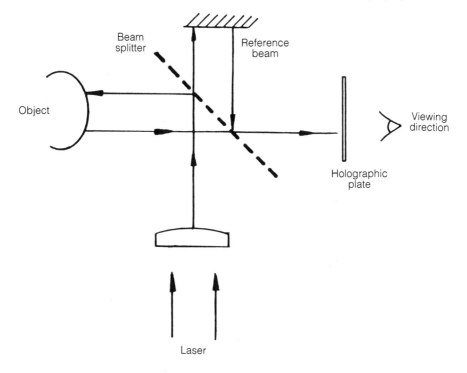

Figure 9.2 Viewing and illumination directions of laser coincident.

9.4.1 Zero fringe method

The following equation describes the general case for relating the fringe order to the displacement

$$n \lambda = \Delta \qquad (9.1)$$

where Δ is the change in the optical path length, n is the fringe order and λ is the wavelength of light. If the viewing and illumination direction are the same as shown in Figure 9.2 and the displacement is in the direction of viewing also, then

$$\frac{n\lambda}{2} = u_z \qquad (9.2)$$

where u_z is the out-of-plane displacement. Provided that the object surface is perpendicular to the viewing direction then the out-of-plane displacements can be found directly from the fringe order.

If the line of sight is not in the direction of movement of the object

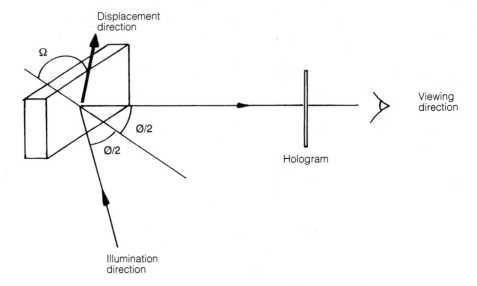

Ω

Displacement
direction

Ø/2

Ø/2

Illumination
direction

Hologram

Viewing
direction

Figure 9.3 Directions of movement, viewing and illumination not coincident.

as shown in Figure 9.3 then the magnitude of the actual displacement is given by:

$$u = \frac{n \lambda}{2 \cos \Omega} \tag{9.3}$$

where Ω is the angle between the line of sight and the direction of the displacement.

If the illumination and viewing directions are not coincident but are at an angle of ϕ then the zero fringe technique gives the component along the bisector of that angle by:

$$u_{\phi/2} = \frac{n \lambda}{2 \cos (\phi/2) \cos \Omega} \tag{9.4}$$

The order of the fringe can only be determined if the zero order fringe is in the field of view. The measurement of absolute displacements also requires knowledge of the geometry of the system which has produced the hologram. However if absolute displacements are not required and it is assumed that only out-of-plane displacements are occurring, the situation is greatly simplified, since the zero order fringe is no longer required. Assuming that the illumination and viewing directions are the same, the difference between the displacements of two points P and Q in the direction of the line of sight, can be found from the absolute displacements of P and Q. If these absolute displacements are u_P and u_Q respectively then:

$$u_P = \frac{n_P\,\lambda}{2} \text{ and } u_Q = \frac{n_Q\,\lambda}{2} \qquad (9.5)$$

where n_P and n_Q are the fringe orders at P and Q.

By subtracting equations (9.5) the difference between the two points gives:

$$u_z = \frac{(n_P - n_Q)\,\lambda}{2} \qquad (9.6)$$

i.e. the displacement of the point P relative to the point Q is the number of fringes between P and Q multiplied by $\lambda/2$.

Therefore, from equation (9.6), it can be seen that out-of-plane displacements are a function of the number of fringes between two points. The higher the density of the fringes, or the narrower the spacing between the fringes, the greater the surface deformation of the specimen. Although the accuracy of this method is high, the main disadvantages are that three separate holograms are needed to complete a full 3-D picture of the deformation, and that the zero order fringe must be identified in order to determine absolute displacements. Double exposure holograms can be interpreted using photographs of the holograms, rather than the holograms themselves.

9.4.2 Fringe counting method

If there is in-plane deformation of the object, then the fringes in the hologram will not, in general, lie on the surface of the object. If an observer looks at a particular object and sweeps the observation from vector position $\mathbf{k}_1$ to $\mathbf{k}_2$ then the number of fringes (Δn) that pass a particular point on the object can be related to the displacement by:

$$\Delta n\,\lambda = \mathbf{u} \cdot (\mathbf{k}_1 - \mathbf{k}_2) \qquad (9.7)$$

where $\mathbf{u}$ is the displacement vector of the object. Simplified forms of this equation can be found for particular circumstances, e.g.

$$u_z = \frac{\Delta n\,\lambda\,L}{d} \qquad (9.8)$$

where L is the distance from the hologram to the reconstructed image and d is the distance scanned, u_z is the out-of-plane displacement (Hewitt, 1982).

This interpretation method can be used for the analysis of components of translation of points in a plane perpendicular to the bisector of the two extremes of the range of sight. The advantages of this technique are that only a single hologram is required to assess all the displacements and no absolute fringe order is required. However the technique has only limited accuracy.

9.5 HOLOGRAPHY IN ORTHOPAEDICS

Holography has been used for analysis of orthopaedic structures for a comparatively short period of time compared to the analysis of other engineering structures and systems. The main areas of interest using holographic interferometry in engineering applications has been for the non-destructive routine analysis of structures such as turbine blades (Erf, 1976), bearing assemblies and also for the testing of aeroplane wing panels (Robinson, 1986). It has been found useful in the detection of faults such as sub-surface or microcrack growth and also for the verification of design intent as a result of the rapid increase in the use of computer models which need to be verified. For large objects and complex assemblies, e.g. aero-engine fans, vibration analysis by holography has been widely carried out and now that high power, double pulsed, ruby lasers have become available the technique is even more versatile.

While much of this general work in the field of holography is of interest, there has also been some interesting work carried out in the field of biomechanics. This has included work using holography for 3-D imagery and surface contouring (Robinson, 1986), however deformation analysis is still the predominant application. The technique has been used to investigate the surface deformations of a variety of orthopaedic systems such as the effect of titanium alloy stems compared with cobalt chromium stems for use in total hip replacements (Manley *et al.*, 1983), on the effect of hip prostheses on the deformation of femora (Hanser, 1979) and in a more detailed study as to the effects of changing the design criteria of the hip prosthesis such as cemented versus cementless, collar contact versus no collar contact on the deformation of the femur (Katz *et al.*, 1990). Other applications have considered the severity of wear on implant materials and devices (Lalor *et al.*, 1971), the transfer of loads across the tibia and fibula and onto the foot (Vukicevic *et al.*, 1979), the deformation of teeth (Matsumoto and Fujita, 1982), an analysis of the deformation of vertebrae under different conditions (Matsumoto *et al.*, 1986) and the behaviour of the plates screwed onto bone across a fracture site (Hanser, 1979; Kojima *et al.*, 1986; Matsumoto *et al.*, 1986; Shelton, 1989; Shelton *et al.*, 1989, 1990). All the investigations were carried out on systems which were extremely difficult to model mathematically because of the complex deformation and strains on the various shaped pieces of bone.

9.6 PRACTICAL HOLOGRAPHIC RECORDING

The holographic apparatus needs to be located in a stable room on a quality vibration isolated table to eliminate vibrations which would produce optical interference of the whole system. A table, such as one with a solid cast iron top and air filled cushions underneath the legs, provides suitable structural and thermal stability. Surrounding the table with curtains helps to reduce draughts which effect the stability of the system and consequently improve the quality and consistency of the holograms. The laser, beam splitter, optical mirrors and collimators can then also be clamped magnetically to the table top. A He–Ne continuous wave (cw) gas laser, wavelength 632.8 nm and nominal power 10 mW can be used for small objects, however for larger objects higher powers are necessary. The most readily available continuous wave lasers are He–Ne lasers, available in power of between 0.01 and 50 mW, and at the top end of the range these lasers have sufficient power, given a stable environment, to record holograms of objects as large as a femur. Argon lasers have slightly lower wavelength, 476–514 nm, and are available at much higher powers (100 mW–15 W) but these are much more expensive, as are He–Cd lasers which have an even lower wavelength of 442–325 nm and are used with an ultraviolet sensitive recording medium.

The beam from the cw laser can be split using a partially reflecting mirror and the object beam is then made divergent by passing it through a collimator. This expanded beam is reflected from the object so that a diffuse wavefront is then incident on the photographic plate. The reference beam is reflected through a series of mirrors and a collimator before falling on the photographic plate. Optical inter-ference and noise, which arise from dust and imperfections in the optics should be removed by passing the reference beam through a spatial filter or pin hole, leaving a clean wave. For the best results the ratio of the object to reference beam intensity should be approximately 1:5 (Jones and Wykes, 1983), which can be achieved by using a variable reflecting mirror and allowing different ratios of light to pass to the reference and object beams depending on the amount of light reflected from the object. The plate holder should be positioned so that the angles of incidence of the reference and object beams are similar. To produce good quality holograms both beams should be adjusted to be the same length within the coherence of the laser, in the case of a He–Ne laser the beams need to be within approximately 5 mm of each other. Suitable glass plates coated with photographic emulsion are supplied by Agfa Gevaert, Belgium, type 8E75AD. These are high sensitivity plates with a grain size of approximately 35 nm, and a resolving power of 5000 lines/mm. The plates are placed with the photographic emulsion facing the incident light.

For a simple approach the plates can be developed in Kodak D–19 developer for 2 min, agitating continuously, washed thoroughly in fresh water and fixed in Iford Hypam fixing solution, diluted in a ratio of 1:4 plus hardener, for a further 1 min. The plates should be washed again thoroughly and left to drip dry. It is possible to bleach these plates, to improve the efficiency of the hologram and hence increase their visibility, by placing them above a beaker containing bromine for a few minutes, then waving them over steam. Alternatively the holograms can be developed, then bleached directly in solutions described by Saxby (1989).

The use of holographic techniques on bone is difficult as bone is not a highly reflective material. The reflectivity is decreased yet further if the bone is wet, as liquid increases the diffraction of the light. The surface of the bone can be sprayed white in order to reduce both these problems. Coating the surface in this way enables the bone to be kept completely wet, while the surface can be wiped dry. This technique makes it possible to record high quality images on small pieces of photographic emulsion coated glass. Increasing the power of the laser also improves the quality of the images. Shorter exposure times can then be used, minimizing the problem of object and optical component movement during the exposure.

Figure 9.4 shows a summary of the fringe patterns which are recorded under standard loading conditions. Figure 9.4 may be used for a more qualitative approach to the problem, essential when the geometry of the surface of the object is unknown or irregular. Qualitatively the technique is extremely sensitive and its main application in many projects has been in the comparison of the different fringe patterns that are produced under different loading conditions. A more quantitative approach to yield accurate measurements of displacement demands three simultaneous holograms, optical analysis followed by a great deal of calculation.

9.7 APPLICATIONS

The results presented in this section show a selection of holograms that have been recorded in various orthopaedic applications.

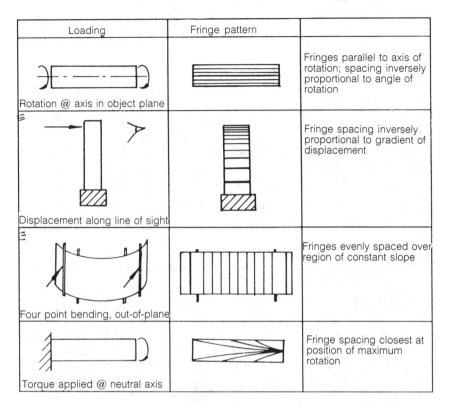

Loading	Fringe pattern	
Rotation @ axis in object plane		Fringes parallel to axis of rotation; spacing inversely proportional to angle of rotation
Displacement along line of sight		Fringe spacing inversely proportional to gradient of displacement
Four point bending, out-of-plane		Fringes evenly spaced over region of constant slope
Torque applied @ neutral axis		Fringe spacing closest at position of maximum rotation

Figure 9.4 Basic holographic fringe patterns produced by different loading conditions.

9.7.1 Fracture fixation

The results presented in Figure 9.5 show the difference between (a) a plate crossing a transverse osteotomy, (b) a plate crossing a 'natural' fracture surface, and (c) a compression plate across an osteotomy site on a human tibia. The holograms were taken of a wet bone, loaded in torsion, rigidly built in on the right hand side, and loaded by applying a dead weight to a lever arm. The technique is sensitive enough to record changes in the fracture configuration – whether the bone ends were in contact or compression had been applied. The discontinuity of fringes in the holograms across the fracture site indicated that a small amount of movement was occurring between the fractured surfaces at small loads. The fringe patterns highlight the need for interdigitation of the bone fragments as this reduces the relative movement of the fracture ends. Compression plates reduce this relative movement still further.

The relative fringe spacing either side of the fracture indicates differ-

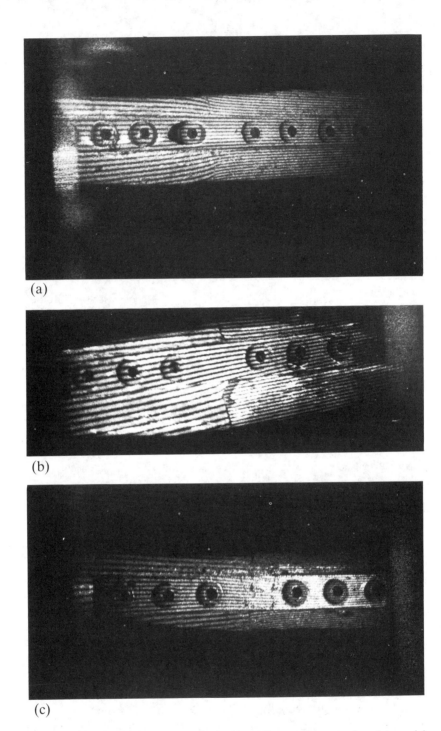

(a)

(b)

(c)

Figure 9.5 (a) Transverse osteotomy fixed with an Osteo self-compression plate applying compression across the fracture site; (b) natural fracture fixed with a stainless steel rectangular plate; (c) transverse osteotomy fixed with a stainless steel rectangular plate.

ent rotations and this is important as interfragmentary movement influences the healing pattern of cortical bone (Hutzschenreuter *et al.*, 1969). The assumption is made in rigid fracture fixation that absolute immobilization of the fracture ends occurs and hence direct or primary bone healing takes place. It is clear from these highly sensitive measurements using holography that complete immobilization is not in fact occurring even when compression is applied across the bone ends as in Figure 9.5(c).

9.7.2 Hip replacement

The hip prostheses were loaded in compression at physiological angles, with a static load of 11.4 N and an additional load of 3.1 N. Holographic interferograms of the posterior aspect of the femur are shown in Figure 9.6. Figure 9.6(a) shows the intact femur, Figure 9.6(b) a Norwich cementless implant without collar contact, and Figure 9.6(c) a Norwich cementless implant with good collar contact. The photographs show a cross-over point indicating the position of maximum displacement of the femur under bending.

The angle of the proximal fringes in Figure 9.6(a) indicate a combination of bending and twisting. On implantation, the fringes are angled more vertically, implying that the deformation is primarily bending with reduced twisting. The fringe pattern is altered from the natural case for the implant with no collar contact (Katz *et al.*, 1990).

9.7.3 Modulus matching

The use of materials that have a higher modulus than bone is universal in orthopaedics. It is felt that this is a problem in several applications, for example, the fibrous encapsulation of screws could be a result of micromovement at the screw–bone interface resulting from the loading of the bone as well as the movement resulting from the loading of the screw. The results presented in Figure 9.7 show the effect of the modulus mismatch for plugs of stainless steel and hydroxyapatite reinforced polyethylene in plaques of bovine bone (Shelton *et al.*, 1990a). The modulus matched implant clearly deforms in a similar manner to bone and shear strains are therefore reduced at the bone implant interface.

9.8 CONCLUSIONS

Holographic interferometry has been found, in many applications, to be a useful method for the analysis of complex systems. It has been shown to provide an overall, full-field view of the whole system, which

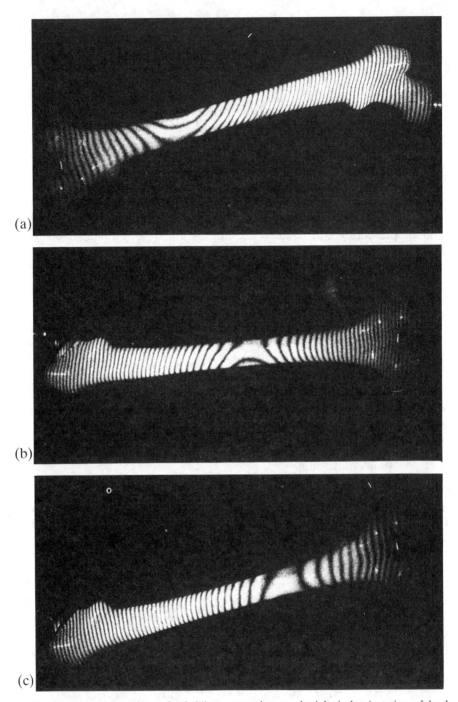

Figure 9.6 (a) Intact femur loaded in compression at physiological orientation of load applied at toe off; (b) femur at same orientation and load with a cementless Norwich total hip replacement inserted without collar contact; (c) same joint replacement with collar contact applied.

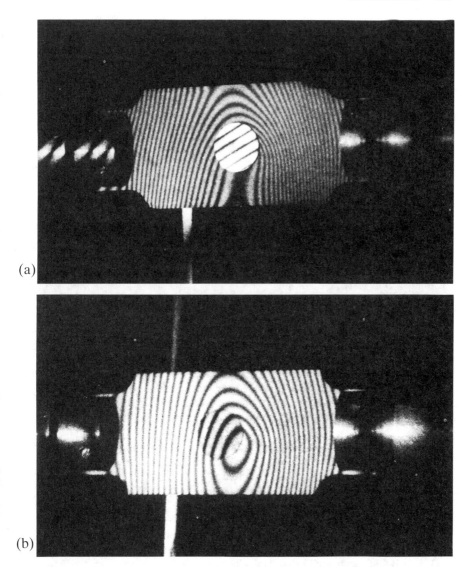

Figure 9.7 A comparison of two materials used as closely fitting plugs in bovine bone with torsion applied: (a) stainless steel; (b) hydroxyapatite reinforced polyethylene.

has, in turn, allowed new features to be observed. Clearly the application for this particular technique has to be carefully chosen due to the problems associated with its sensitivity. However once a suitable project has been identified, the technique allows the overall performance of a system or structure to be analysed in a unique manner at extremely high sensitivity.

REFERENCES

Abramson, N. (1974) Sandwich hologram interferometry: a new dimension in holographic comparison. *Appl. Optics*, **13**, 2019–25.

Abramson, N. (1981) *The Making and Evaluation of Holograms*, Academic Press, New York, London.

Briers, J., (1976) Review, the interpretation of holographic interferograms. *Opt. Quant. Electron.*, **8**, 469–501.

Erf, R. (1974) *Holographic Nondestructive Testing*, Academic Press, New York, London.

Gabor, D. (1948) A new microscopic principle. *Nature*, **161**, 777–8.

Hanser, U. (1979) Quantitative evaluation of holographic deformation investigations in experimental orthopaedics, in *Holography in Medicine and Biology* (ed. G. von Bally), Springer-Verlag, Heidelburg.

Hewitt, A. (1982) Holographic studies of bone response to small forces, PhD thesis, University of London.

Hutzschenreuter, P., Steinemann, S., Perren, S.M., Geret, M. and Klebl, M. (1969) Some effects of rigidity of internal fixation on healing patterns of osteotomies. *Injury*, **1**, 77–82.

Jones, R. and Wykes, C. (1983) *Holographic and Speckle Interferometry*, Cambridge University Press, Cambridge.

Katz, D., Tanner, K.E. and Bonfield, W. (1990) A biomechanical analysis of the implanted human femur using holography. *Abstracts of European Society of Biomechanics*, Aarhus, Denmark, P42.

Kojima, A., Ogawa, R., Izuchi, N., Matsumoto, T., Iwata, K. and Nagata, R. (1986) Holographic investigation of the mechanical properties of tibia fixed with internal fixation plates, in *Biomechanics: Basic and Applied Research* (eds G. Bergmann, R. Kölbel and A. Rohlmann), Martinus Nijhoff, Dordrecht, pp. 243–8.

Lalor, M.J., Groves, D. and Atkinson, J.T. (1971) Holographic studies of wear in implant materials and devices, in *Holography in Medicine and Biology* (ed. G. von Bally), Springer-Verlag, Heidelburg.

Manley, M.T., Gurtowski, J., Stern, L., Halioa, M. and Bowlins, T. (1983) A biomechanical study of the proximal femur using fullfield holographic interferometry. *Trans. Orthop. Res. Soc.*, **29**, 99.

Matsumoto, T. and Fujita, T. (1982) Holographic interferometry of tooth deformations, *Optics in Biomedical Sciences Proc. of Int. Conf.*, Graz, Austria (ed. G. von Bally), Springer-Verlag, Heidelburg.

Matsumoto, T., Kojima, A., Ogawa, R., Iwata, K. and Nagata, R. (1986) Deformation measurement of lumbar vertebra by holographic interferometry. *Int. Conf. on Holographic Applications*, China.

Piwernetz, K. (1979) Holography in orthopaedics, in *Holography in Medicine and Biology* (ed. G. von Bally), Springer-Verlag, Heidelburg.

Robinson, D.W. (1986) Holography edges closer to the shop floor. *Chartered Mech. Enger.*, **33**, 36–40.

Saxby, G. (1989) *Practical Holography*, Prentice Hall, New York.

Shelton, J.C. (1989) Stability and failure of internal fracture fixation plates, PhD thesis, University of London.

Shelton, J.C., Gorman, D. and Bonfield, W. (1989) Double exposure holographic interferometric evaluation of plated fracture systems. *Proc. XII Int. Congress of Biomech.*, Los Angeles, USA, abstract 61, International Society of Biomechanics.

Shelton, J.C., Gorman, D. and Bonfield, W. (1990) Application of holographic interferometry to investigate internal fracture fixations plates. *J. Mater. Sci. Mater. Med.*, **1**, 146–53.

Vest, C.M. (1979) *Holographic Interferometry*, John Wiley, New York.

von Bally, G. (1979) *Holography in Medicine and Biology*, Springer-Verlag, Heidelburg.

Vukicevic, D., Nikolic, V., Vukicevic, S., Hancevic, J. and Sucur, Z. (1979) Holographic investigation of the mechanical characteristics of the complex foot in conditions of lesion and reconstruction, in *Holography in Medicine and Biology* (ed. G. von Bally), Springer-Verlag, Heidelburg.

10

Strain measurement by thermoelastic emission

J.L. Duncan

10.1 INTRODUCTION

The phenomenon of thermoelastic emission, that is heating of the material due to the elastic work of deformation, was first described by Lord Kelvin in 1878 (Thomson, 1878) but could not be implemented at that time due to the lack of sufficiently high resolution thermal detectors. The deformation induced change in temperature is proportional to the sum of the principal stresses when there is no heat transfer, that is under adiabatic conditions. The necessary infra-red detectors to measure such thermal emissions have become available in recent years and permitted the development of the SPATE (Stress Pattern Analysis by Thermal Emission) system for full-field experimental stress analysis (Mountain and Weber, 1978). This equipment is based on a scanning radiometer which measures the slight temperature changes produced on the surface of a structure which is undergoing cycle loading.

The thermodynamic relationship (Biot, 1956) between these temperature changes and the corresponding stresses produced by the applied load is used to determine either the full-field surface stress distribution or that along a line on the specimen.

$$\Delta T = \frac{-\alpha \, T \, \Delta\sigma}{\rho \, C_\sigma} \tag{10.1}$$

where ΔT is the change in temperature, α is the linear coefficient of expansion, T is the absolute temperature of the structure, $\Delta\sigma$ is the sum of the principal stresses, ρ is the material density and C_σ is the specific heat at constant stress. Thus tension leads to cooling and compression to heating in most materials. Jordon and Sandor (1978) have verified this relationship experimentally.

10.2 DESCRIPTION OF SPATE SYSTEM

The system consists of a computer controlled non-contacting infra-red detector which uses mirrors to scan over the surface of the object of interest while it is undergoing cyclic loading. This can be used either to produce a full-field colour contour map, showing the magnitude and distribution of the sum of the principal stresses over visible surfaces on the structure subjected to dynamic loading or, to give a scan along a line on the surface of the structure. A colour monitor is used to display a false colour image of the stress levels over the scanned area.

If a suitable calibration has been performed qualitative stress levels are displayed; quantitative or relative values of stress are shown if no calibration factors have been incorporated and are indicated by a 16 level colour scale which is displayed adjacent to the thermoelastic stress patterns. Calibration may be theoretical using the known properties of the material, which may be substituted into equation (10.1) but sufficiently precise data can be difficult to obtain and other factors need to be taken into account to give the full equation

$$\Delta\sigma = \frac{-D \ V \ R \ \rho \ C_{\mathrm{p}}}{\alpha \ T \ e} \tag{10.2}$$

where D is responsivity of the detector, V is amplitude of the thermo-elastic response voltage, R is a correction factor for temperature changes in wavelength and radiation intensity and e is the surface emissivity of the material being scanned. Thus it is advantageous to perform the calibration with an external mechanism. This is done either by using a standard shaped piece of bone and by applying known loads so that known stresses are produced or with strain gauges. The latter is difficult with bone as the conversion from strains to the sum of the principal stresses requires knowledge of the Young's moduli and Poisson's ratios of the bone being studied.

The heart of the system is a highly sensitive infra-red detector and an amplifier/analyser which generates a signal in response to the thermoelastic flux emitted from a spot on the surface of the structure which is undergoing uniform cyclic loading. A germanium lens in conjunction with computer controlled motorized horizontal and vertical scanning mirrors focuses the thermoelastic flux from the object surface on to the infra-red detector. The depth of focus of the system is such that the system is not restricted to flat surfaces but may be used on complex three-dimensional surfaces. In addition to the detector signal a reference signal, derived either from the test machine signal generator or from the test machine load cell, is applied to the SPATE analyser to allow the phase relationship between the response and reference signals to be determined. This phase relationship indicates whether the stress is tensile or compressive. The collected and digitized data can either be stored on a floppy disk or down loaded onto a mainframe or minicomputer for further analysis.

The instrument sensitivity is 0.001 K, which equates to stress levels of 1 MPa in steels and 0.4 MPa in aluminium. To exclude thermal changes due to heat conduction a sufficiently high rate of loading is required and the minimum practical rate is 3 Hz. Normal ambient temperature variations do not dominate the thermoelastic output since these changes do not occur at the same frequency as the load reference signal and are therefore rejected by the signal analyser.

The detector in this system functions under cryogenic conditions and therefore must be maintained at low temperature by cooling with liquid nitrogen ($-196°C$). A visible light beam aligned with the optical axis of the lens allows the operator to select any point on the specimen for individual measurement or to set the limits of the scan field or of a line scan. SPATE uses infra-red signals with wavelengths of 8–13 μm and at these wavelengths oxygen and nitrogen are low energy absorbers. Although carbon dioxide and water vapour do absorb slightly more energy, at less than 10 m range this absorption is probably insignificant unless there are very high levels of these gases (Duncan, 1988).

The advantages of SPATE are that it uses the real object rather than a model, high resolution scans of full-field stress patterns may be obtained either quantitatively or qualitatively, and good spatial resolution (0.5 mm) may be obtained over large areas (greater than 1 m²), for larger areas the spatial resolution is reduced. Complex geometries may be investigated. Minimal surface preparation is required other than cleaning to remove the soft tissue, as this is not highly stressed, and spraying with a high emissivity paint, if the material has low emissivity, allows high sensitivity to stress to be achieved. The disadvantages include the inability to investigate static stresses and this includes plastic deformation as if the elastic limit is exceeded these deformations produce isothermal rather than adiabatic temperature changes (Harwood and Cummings, 1986, 1991). In rough areas of bone, like the linea aspera on the posterior aspect of the femur, the bone cannot be sufficiently well cleaned to produce a good signal. The pattern obtained is the sum of the principal stresses and thus pure shear stresses lead to zero output as has been verified by Stanley and Chan (1985). Only surface stresses may be studied but these reflect the internal stresses, geometry and elastic moduli. Calibration is straightforward for standard isotropic materials; with anisotropic materials, including bone, this is more difficult. It should also be noted that the system is very expensive.

10.3 EXPERIMENTAL WORK USING SPATE

Early experiments at the National Engineering Laboratory (Duncan, 1988) used whole bovine tibiae and prepared specimens of bovine tibia; a Brazilian disk, that is a disk loaded along a diagonal, and a hole in plate specimen loaded with 0.6 ± 0.5 kN at a frequency of 6 Hz, showed that bone produced sufficient thermal output to be detected by the SPATE system and that the resulting stress patterns shown in Figure 10.1 were similar to those predicted by elastic theory. This encouraged the testing of more complex specimens.

A fresh proximal section of human femur was cleaned of all soft tissue and periosteum with the exception of the abductor muscle attachment to the greater trochanter. The distal end of the femur was embedded in acrylic cement in a metal sleeve in the normal physiological orientation. A cup to represent the acetabulum was used to apply load to the femoral head and surgical cord was woven into the abductor ligaments to allow the attachment, via a flexible belt, to a second actuator representing the abductor muscles. The complete experimental arrangement is shown in Figure 10.2.

The technique requires that the applied load be dynamic in character to ensure that adiabatic conditions apply within the test material. Therefore some consideration must be given to both the range of applied load and to the frequency of application in order that any viscoelastic effects are negligible. The loads chosen in these particular experiments were sinusoidal, 1.0 ± 0.8 kN for the femoral head load and 0–0.4 kN for the trochanteric load and the frequency was 6 Hz.

This loading regime was considered to be a reasonable compromise between the length of time required for a high resolution SPATE scan and a sufficiently low rate of strain to ensure insignificant viscoelastic effects (Bonfield and Clark, 1973; Huiskes, 1987). An estimate of the strain rate for these loading conditions and the particular femur used in the experiment, measured in the region of high stress in the proximal medial femur, was 4000 $\mu\epsilon$ s^{-1} similar to the maximum physiological strain rates of 4000 $\mu\epsilon$ s^{-1} measured by Lanyon *et al.* (1975) on the human tibia in walking.

A series of four medium resolution scans in steps of 90° were taken of the loaded natural femur to determine the areas and viewing directions of interest. An example of such a scan, taken from an anterior viewpoint, is shown in Figure 10.3. This shows an area of relatively high stress in the region of the medial proximal femur diminishing quickly to a nominally even value of stress along the remainder of the femoral shaft. As has been suggested by Cowin (1987), the stress levels along a bone should be constant along the long axis as the theories of bone remodelling suggest that the bone will remodel to constant stress

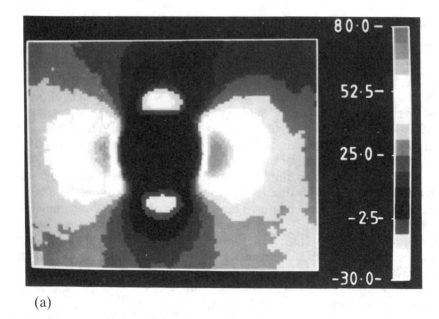

(a)

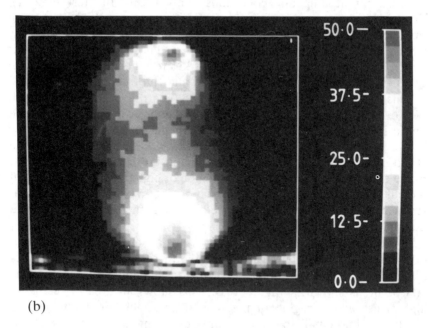

(b)

Figure 10.1 (a) Full field SPATE pattern generated by compressive loading of a Hole in Plate specimen machined from a bovine tibia; (b) full field SPATE pattern generated by compressive loading of a Brazilian disk specimen of bovine bone with the long axis of the bone vertical.

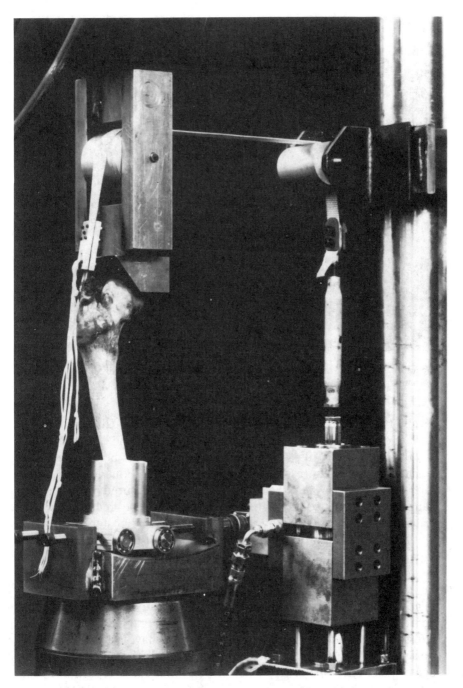

Figure 10.2 Mechanical set-up for testing a proximal section of femur by applying a compressive load to the femoral head and a tensile load to the hip abductor mechanicsm.

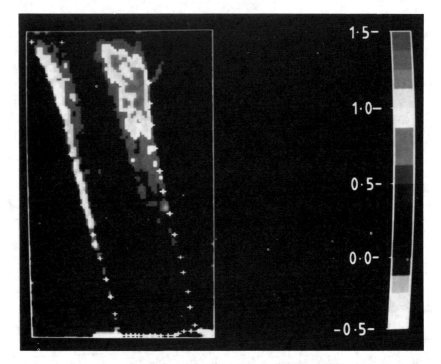

Figure 10.3 SPATE scan of the anterior view of a natural femur distal to the greater trochanter loaded through the femoral head and the greater trochanter.

levels. It should be noted that along the midline the false colours are dark and thus appear to be zero when actually they lie between -1.25×10^2 and 3.75×10^2 MPa. The high stress levels below the lesser trochanter are of interest as this is an area of thin bone leading to the high stress levels when the strain values as measured with a strain gauge would not be as high, and would also be reduced by the reinforcement of the bone by the strain gauge. The posterior scan was ignored due to the problem of removing the soft tissue from the linea aspera.

Another feature of the SPATE system is that selected line scans can be taken between two fixed points on the surface. This has the advantage that a stress profile can be obtained in relatively short time compared to a full-field scan and displays a simple graphic distribution of stress along the defined line. These line scans have a lower signal-to-noise ratio in general than the normalized full-field scans and an average or peak envelope of stress has to be estimated. A typical line scan taken in the high stressed region is shown after smoothing in Figure 10.4.

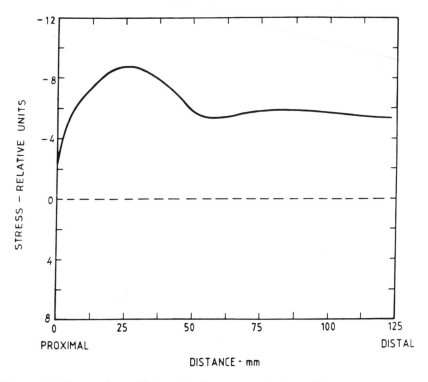

Figure 10.4 Line scan from mid-line of the femur shown in Figure 10.3.

A commercially available stainless steel femoral stem was inserted into the femur using the standard surgical technique giving calcar contact and fixed using conventional polymethylmethacrylate bone cement. The original test arrangement was modified so that the matching high molecular weight polyethylene acetabular cup was incorporated in the test rig to apply load to the head of the prosthesis.

SPATE scans, both full-field and line, were taken from the same viewing angles and with identical loading conditions as in Figure 10.3. The resulting full-field and line scans are shown in Figures 10.5 and 10.6. Comparison of the full-field scans in Figures 10.3 and 10.5, making allowance for the change in the stress levels related to any particular colour value, show the removal of the stress concentration below the lesser trochanter as this area is reinforced by the implant and the bone cement. The tensile stress levels along the lateral aspect of the femur are increased and the compressive stress levels are decreased. The line scans, Figures 10.4 and 10.6, indicate that the introduction of a metallic femoral stem markedly reduces the stress levels on the proximal femur.

The results obtained are comparable with the qualitative results

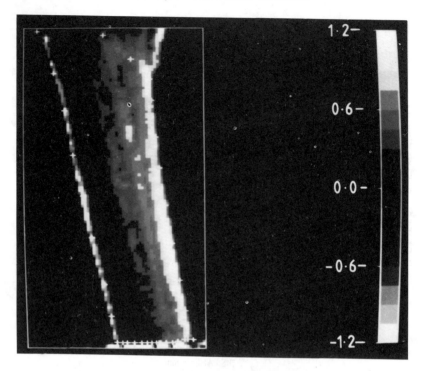

Figure 10.5 SPATE scan of the anterior view of a femur distal to the greater trochanter after replacement with a cemented femoral component and loaded through the femoral head and the greater trochanter.

obtained by other methods, i.e. strain gauges and finite element analysis (Rohlmann *et al.*, 1982, 1983) and are shown in Figure 10.7.

10.4 DISCUSSION

The method of determining stress distribution on fresh bone using a thermoelastic technique appears to be consistent with conventional elastic theory and with other techniques used to determine stress and strain distributions in materials. The method may therefore be used at this stage of its development for initial surveys of stress/strain distributions in its own right, or may be used in conjunction with other techniques either for verification or model refinement.

As with any other method of stress analysis there are advantages and disadvantages in using the thermoelastic method. The advantages are that a real bone is used for the stress analysis and therefore there is no requirement for complex modelling, assumptions of geometry or load transfer across interfaces. There is no preparation required of the

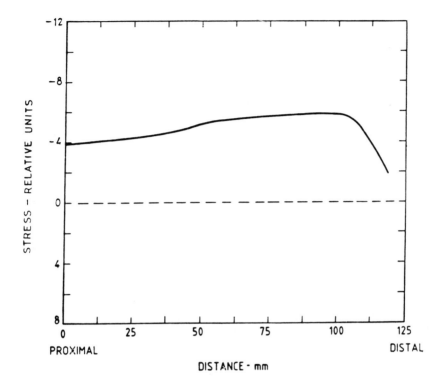

Figure 10.6 Line scan from the mid-line of a femur after replacement with a cemented femoral component, loaded as in Figure 10.5.

bone other than that it should be free of all soft tissue and that the surface is dry during scanning.

The disadvantages are mainly those to be expected when dealing with biological material, namely material degradation and biological hazard. These disadvantages may be minimized by cold storage (−20°C) of the bone tissue when not in use, with the provision that sufficient time is allowed for thawing and that during thawing the bone is wrapped in a saline soaked cloth to prevent drying which will effect the behaviour of the bone. The cold storage method has minimal effect on the mechanical properties of bone (Sedlin and Hirsch, 1966). Normal clinical precautions should be taken to prevent any biological hazard.

The stress patterns obtained by SPATE in both the Brazilian disks and hole-in-plate experiments did not show the marked effect of anisotropy that would be expected from a material such as bone. Experiments conducted on two types of wood, teak and beech, showed marked elongation of the stress patterns along the high modulus axis, but the ratio of the Young's moduli for these materials is greater than

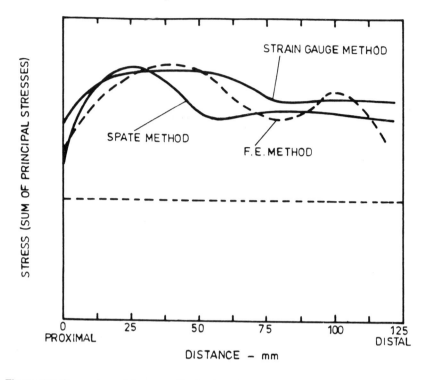

Figure 10.7 Comparison of the stress distributions along natural femora obtained by SPATE and finite element and strain gauging from the data of Rohlmann *et al.* (1982, 1983).

that of bone. More specific measurements on specimens of known properties are necessary to solve this problem.

The full-field scans of the proximal femur show an edge effect, this is thought to be due to movement of the femur in the direction perpendicular to the viewing axis so that the edge points move in and out of certain pixels on the detector giving readings which are sums of background noise and the heat generated by the stress. Motion parallel to the optic axis does not have this effect.

A suggestion by Huiskes (1987) that if only the maximum principal stresses (or equivalents stresses) are of interest the femoral diaphysis can in all loading conditions, except that of torsion, be considered as a linear isotropic and homogeneous solid, a good accuracy in stress analysis may be obtained, since the stress patterns obtained by SPATE are the result of the sum of the principal stresses and therefore under the Huiskes criteria would result in a stress pattern which would appear to originate from an essentially isotropic material and thus resolve the problem obtained from the Brazilian disk and hole-in-plate specimens. A theoretical treatment of the thermoelastic stress analysis of fibre composites (Potter and Greaves, 1987) may give further insight into the effects of anistropy on SPATE stress patterns.

10.5 CONCLUSIONS

SPATE has been shown to give a good full-field view of the stress levels in bone and how these are altered by insertion of an implant. It is non-contacting, requires little preparation of the specimen and may be used for complex shapes like the femur and the pelvis. It is however expensive and it may be argued that the loading rates are higher than physiological.

REFERENCES

Biot, M.A. (1956) Thermoelasticity and irreversible thermodynamics. *J. Appl. Phys.*, **27**, 240–53.

Bonfield, W. and Clark, E.A. (1973) Elastic deformation of compact bone. *J. Mater. Sci.*, **8**, 1590–4.

Cowin, S.C. (1987) The mechanical and stress adaptive properties of bone. *Ann. Biomed. Engng.*, **11**, 263–95.

Duncan, J.L. (1988) A method of stress analysis on fresh bone by thermoelastic emission, PhD thesis, University of Strathclyde, Glasgow, Scotland.

Harwood, N. and Cummings, W.M. (1986) Applications of thermoelastic stress analysis. *Strain*, **22** (1), 7–12.

Harwood, N. and Cummings, W.M. (1991) *Thermoelastic Stress Analysis*, Adam Hilger, Bristol, UK.

Huiskes, R. (1987) Communication to delegates. *Conference on Bone Mechanics*, Urdine, Italy, July 1987.

Jordon, E.H. and Sandor, B.I. (1978) Stress analysis from temperature data. *J. Stress Anal.*, **6**, 325–31.

Lanyon, L.E., Hampson,W.G.J., Goodship, A.E. and Shah, J.S. (1975) Bone deformation recorded *in vivo* from strain gauges attached to the human tibial shaft. *Acta Orthop. Scand.*, **46**, 256–68.,

Mountain, D.S. and Weber, J.M.B. (1978) Stress pattern analysis by thermal emission. *Proc. Soc. Photo-Optic. Instr. Engng*, **164**, 189–96.

Potter, R.T. and Greaves, L.J. (1987) The application of thermoelastic stress techniques to fibre composites. *Proc. Photo-Optic. Instr. Engng.*, **819**, 134–41.

Rohlmann, A., Mossner, U.. and Bergmann, G. (1983) Finite element analysis and experimental investigation in a femur with a total hip endo-prosthesis. *J. Biomech.*, **16**, 727–42.

Rohlmann, A., Mossner, U., Bergmann, G. and Kölbel, R. (1982) Finite element analysis and experimental investigation of stresses in a femur. *J. Biomed. Engng.*, **4**, 241–6.

Sedlin, E.D. and Hirsch, C. (1966) Factors affecting the determination of the physical properties of femoral cortical bone. *Acta Orthop. Scand.*, **37**, 29–48.

Stanley, P. and Chan, W.K. (1985) Stress analysis by means of the thermoelastic effect. *J. Strain Anal.*, **20**, 129–37.

Thomson, W. (Lord Kelvin) (1878) On the thermoelastic, thermomagnetic and pyroelectric properties of matter. *Phil. Mag.*, **5**, 4–27.

11

Modelling for stress analysis in biomechanics

A.L. Yettram

11.1 INTRODUCTION

Apart from its many other functions, the human body is both a mechanism (it transmits movement) and a structure (it transmits force). As a structure, its elements suffer mechanical stress and consequently mechanical strain. Over many years efforts have been made to analyse theoretically the structural behaviour of components of the human and animal anatomy when subjected to force. The methods used have been those available at the time applied to the contemporary theories of stress and structural analysis. The work has been carried out by investigators from many disciplines – biologists, clinicians, physicists and, of course, engineers. A perusal of the literature in this field shows that there are virtually no parts of the human body which have escaped the attention of analysts. Hard, and obviously load-bearing, structures such as bone and cartilage, have attracted much of this attention, but so also have soft tissues such as those involved in the cardiovascular system. This book is primarily devoted to experimental determinations of strain. These experimental techniques are, however, expensive and time consuming to apply. While the importance of experimental data is paramount, the potential for numerical approaches such as finite-element methods to complement experimental studies is very great. This can be achieved in a number of significant ways; analytical methods can be used to evaluate parametric changes to signal major influences and to assist in improved design of experiments. There have been significant advances made in finite element studies in recent years and the technique is gaining even greater credibility in the field of biomechanics all the more because of its application in parallel with experimental work. In this chapter only one anatomical component will be considered in detail – the proximal end of the human femur both in its entire state and also when modified by the implementation of a total hip replacement – to illustrate the role of modelling in biomechanics.

11.2 SOME BASIC CONCEPTS

Before dealing with a specific application it is apposite to consider the principles which underlie the science and art of structural and stress analysis itself. Complex structures, whether of an engineering kind such as bridges or aircraft, or of a natural or biological kind such as the human musculo-skeletal system, consist of interconnected components. As a whole they may be acted upon by external forces and/or displacements, but living structures differ from inert engineering structures in that they include elements, muscles, which themselves generate force. The determination of the interactive internal forces which affect the structural elements might be called 'structural' analysis whereas the detailed determination of how these forces are distributed as stresses within the elements could be described as 'stress' analysis.

The basic problem of stress or structural analysis can be succinctly expressed with reference to Figure 11.1, which might be called 'the structural chain'. The four parameters involved are force, stress, strain and displacement. They are connected in pairs by three links: equilibrium (involving force and stress), mechanical properties (relating stress and strain) and compatibility (involving strain and displacement). Equilibrium and compatibility are conditions imposed by the laws of mechanics, while for any particular material the nature of the mechanical properties link is determined experimentally. In any real structural problem the applied forces and displacements are such that some of each are known *ab initio* (actions) and the rest are unknown initially (reactions). Where a force is known its displacement is unknown whilst where a displacement is known the corresponding force is unknown. Stress and strain are internal effects and are all unknown initially. What ensures that a structure (which is stable, i.e. the laws of equilibrium are satisfied and remains in a compatible state, i.e. the laws of compatibility are satisfied) will behave in a unique manner which can be solved analytically, is that there always exists a known displacement corresponding to an unknown force and vice versa.

That this is so is true in theory; in practice things are not so simple. This is because a structure comprises an infinity of points on the

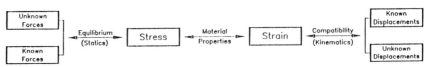

Figure 11.1 The structural chain.

boundary where forces act and displacements occur and in the interior where stress and strain exist. The situation is somewhat akin to having an infinite number of simultaneous equations in an infinity of unknowns – there may well be a unique solution set but it cannot be obtained with a finite amount of effort. Stress and structural analysis can be approached from either end of the structural chain depending upon whether the unknown forces or the unknown displacements are considered the primary unknowns. If the former is the case the approach is known as a force (or flexibility) method whereas for the latter the approach is known as the displacement (or stiffness) method. When the force method is adopted the situation is considered as a structure which is effectively statically indeterminate whereas when approached from the displacement method point of view the system is considered as a mechanism which is kinematically indeterminate.

Thus any realistic structure is indeterminate to the infinite degree. In order to reduce a problem to a finite degree of indeterminacy so that a solution can be obtained, approximations, idealizations or assumptions, and other simplifications have to be introduced. These can take many forms and the more common ones may be listed conveniently under the following headings:

1. Geometry: the physical shape of the body may be assumed to be simpler than it is in reality.
2. Material properties: the physical behaviour of materials and their various mechanical properties, such as elasticity, viscoelasticity, plasticity, may be assumed to be simpler than they really are.
3. The form of the material properties: inhomogeneity or anisotropy of material properties may be ignored in order to simplify analysis.
4. The distribution of the material of the structure: the actual continuous nature of the material within a structure may be considered rearranged to simplify modelling.
5. The boundary conditions: the loading and restraint conditions may be considered simpler than they are in reality, for example by invoking St Venant's Principle.
6. The form of the solution: the form of a solution, if not its absolute value, can be arbitrarily assumed, say from previous experience.
7. The mathematics: the mathematics used to arrive at a solution from the data may introduce approximations.

In the general field of engineering stress and structural analysis many of the simplifications referred to are used in the modelling process. This will depend both upon how well the physical properties of a structure are known and also upon how important is the accuracy of the solution relative to the amount of analytical and computational effort required. The 'art' element in stress analysis is to find the most satisfactory solution with the minimum amount of effort.

11.3 APPLICATION TO BIOMECHANICS

In conventional engineering very accurate solutions can be obtained very efficiently especially using modern computer aids to perform the calculations required. In biomechanical stress analysis the situation is much more difficult. Just to obtain the basic physical data required in a model, the geometry, the material properties and the boundary conditions, presents a great challenge. From the point of view of modelling, biological and anatomical structures are of arbitrary shape that differ between individuals and are of course also dependent on the age of the subject. Models can be reconstructed from data obtained by medical imaging of patients *in vivo* although not with the precision that measurements can be made from cadaveric tissue. Obtaining a realistic description of the mechanical properties of tissues is a far more difficult problem. The normal techniques of experimentation to obtain tissue compliances can only be applied to *in vitro* specimens, and a great deal of work has been done in this way on many of the tissues of the body to obtain their stress/strain characteristics. However, living tissues can behave differently from their dead counterparts, for example by their compliance being affected by the pressures within the fluids which they contain. An account of tissue stiffnesses and flexibilities will be found elsewhere in texts dealing with the mechanical properties of such tissues (Yamada, 1970; Fung, 1981). The human, and animal body also differ, from the engineering structure in that they contain structural elements which are both passive and active. Muscles are essential structural components of the body in that they can carry load, but they also are living and therefore actively create tensile forces. Thus if part of the anatomy is isolated as a free body the forces to which it may be subjected are not necessarily only from external sources, or from self-weight, but may also arise from the contained musculature as discussed in Chapter 2. In the musculo-skeletal system calculation of the distribution of forces is a special case of structural analysis which, because of the active components, involves techniques which are not required in conventional engineering. As has been mentioned earlier, theoretical stress and structural analysis techniques have been applied to most parts of the human anatomy both in its natural state and when including artificial implants. This has been done for many reasons – for the acquisition of basic anatomical knowledge, for clinical and diagnostic purposes and for assisting in the design of tissue replacements. In the context of the present chapter attention will be paid here to merely one particular component – the human femur and in particular the modification to its proximal end arising from the need for hip replacement.

11.3.1 The intact femur

Considering the intact femur as a typical unidimensional member, i.e. one in which the length is much greater than any cross-section dimension, in some of the early work on its structural behaviour it was treated according to the Engineers Theory of Bending allied with the St Venant Torsion Theory. Typical are the analyses of Toridis (1969) and of Piotrowski and Wilcox (1971). The same approach has been presented more recently by Raftopoulos and Qassem (1987) who have taken into account the curvature of the femur and the anisotropy of its material as well as there being both cortical and cancellous bone present. Rybicki *et al.* (1972) also applied beam theory to the full femur but pointed out that the results were only meaningful in the mid-shaft region. At the ends, the epiphyses, a more sophisticated method was called for and they modelled these areas using the finite-element method. This was one of the earliest applications of this method to biological structures. There are many textbooks now available on finite-element analysis (Nath, 1974; Gallagher *et al.*, 1982; Zienkiewicz, 1989) and with the development of computing equipment its use has become commonplace in all stress analyses. This is particularly so with the current availability of user-friendly packages. Its attraction in the biomechanics field is its ability to deal with non-homogeneous structures of irregular geometry. The most important aspect of the application of the finite element method is in the initial modelling of the real system. This is very much down to the skill and experience of the analyst (NAFEMS, 1986).

In the work of Rybicki *et al.* (1972) the diaphysis of the femur was modelled as a two-dimensional plate of elements assigned varying degrees of stiffness to compensate for the thickness variation of the actual bone. Brekelmans and Poort (1973) also applied the finite-element method to the full femur at this time, modelling the entire bone rather than just the end regions, but again as a two-dimensional plate. They also assumed the structure to be homogeneous, linear elastic and isotropic, and investigated two configurations, one where the plate was assigned a uniform thickness and a second, which they referred to as 'semi-three-dimensional' where the thickness was varied to accord with the real bone. Valliappan *et al.* (1977) modelled the proximal femur using three-dimensional eight-noded isoparametric elements (Figure 11.2). They progressively refined the mesh used until convergence of the results was obtained. In their model they differentiated the regions of cancellous and cortical bone. Rohlmann *et al.*

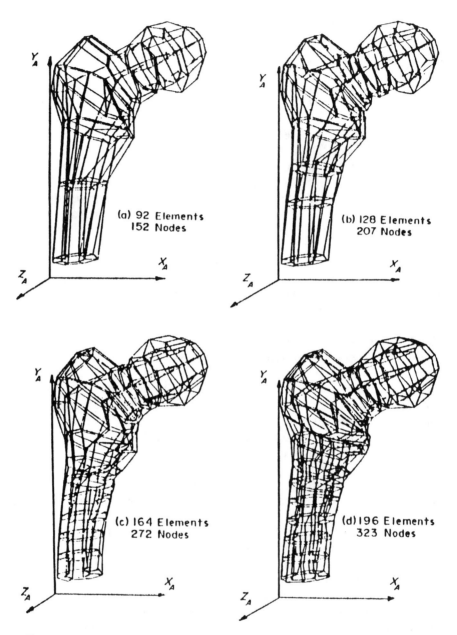

Figure 11.2 Progressive refinement of a mesh for the analysis of the proximal end of a full femur (from Valliappan *et al.*, *Comp. Biol. Med.*, **7**, 258; reproduced by permission of Pergamon Press).

(1982) presented a quite detailed three-dimensional finite element model of virtually a complete femur. They also used eight-noded hexahedral elements, 1950 in number giving rise to 7188 degrees of freedom, and took both cortical and cancellous bone into account although considering both of them as isotropic and linearly elastic.

Apart from the analyses referred to above where the interest was mainly in consideration of the structural capabilities of the femur, more recent work in this area has also been carried out to shed light on the relationship between the form of the bone and biological effects. Brown *et al.* (1980), for example, carried out plane strain analyses of a coronal mid-section of the proximal femur using quadratic finite elements in their model. The cancellous bone was treated as anisotropic and non-homogeneous and their study was concerned with the effect of regions of aseptic necrosis being present. This was considered by varying the stiffnesses of the elements representing the infarcted region and noting the changes in patterns of stress distribution which ensued. Carter *et al.* (1989) also developed a plane strain model of the proximal femur, in this case to study correlations between stress distribution and the trabecular architecture of the cancellous bone. This was carried out using an iterative procedure where material properties of elements were changed depending upon the stresses generated in each iterative cycle. They also performed similar work (Fyhrie and Carter, 1990) with particular emphasis on the relationship between cancellous bone density and stress, but this time using an axisymmetric idealization of the head of the femur modelled with eight-noded brick elements.

11.3.2 The implanted femur

Turning now to the situation of the composite structure consisting of an implanted femoral component of a total hip replacement, some early attempts at analysis were made which called upon beam theory. For example Gola and Gugliotta (1979) devised a simplified two-dimensional coupled beam model to reproduce the linkage between the elements which are interconnected over a common region of their lengths. Bartel and Desormeaux (1977) considered the prosthesis/cement/bone combination as a single composite beam of three elements each with its own flexural rigidity. They compared the results which this model predicted with those from an idealized three-dimensional axisymmetric finite element assemblage. Clearly the complex geometry of a femur with an implanted endoprosthesis, allied to the non-homogeneity of the bone pointed to the use of the finite element method as the most suitable approach and since that time almost all analyses

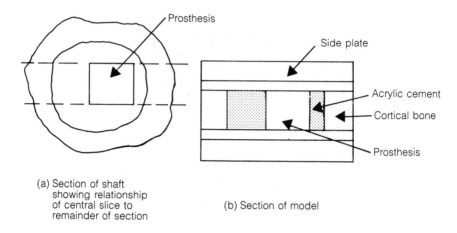

(a) Section of shaft
    showing relationship
    of central slice to   (b) Section of model
    remainder of section

Figure 11.3 (a) Cross-section of femoral cortex, cement, prothesis, with (b) two-dimensional idealization (from Svensson *et al.* (1976)).

have adopted this technique with various degrees of simplification in the model.

McNeice (1975) presented the results from a two-dimensional plane stress model using isoparametric elements whose thicknesses were determined in accordance with the stiffnesses of the relevant materials. A similar model was adopted by Andriacchi *et al.* (1976) but was further developed by this same group (Hampton *et al.*, 1976) to incorporate a 'spanning element' to represent the fact that the medial and lateral aspects of the femoral cortex worked in conjunction with each other as they were essentially both parts of the same 'tubula' component. They also devised a three-dimensional model of the same system. Svensson *et al.* (1976) also used the technique of creating a pseudo two-dimensional model (Figure 11.3) having 'side plates' or 'spanning elements' to compensate for the three-dimensional nature of the system. Anand *et al.* (1978) idealized the mid and proximal regions of an implant as axisymmetric but took into account the non-axisymmetric nature of the loading.

Yettram and Wright (1979) used a two-dimensional plane stress model (Figure 11.4) mainly to examine the effect on the bone cement of varying such parameters as the taper of the prosthesis stem and the stiffness of the prosthesis and cement. In this model, however, the orthotropic nature of the cortical bone was taken into account. It was further used to investigate the stress in the stem itself (Yettram and Wright, 1980).

The availability of progressively more powerful computers is reflected in the move to greater realism in the models analysed by the finite element method. For example Hampton *et al.* (1980) and

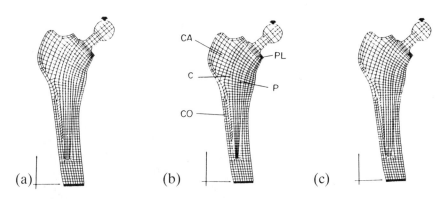

Figure 11.4 Two-dimensional finite element meshes for: (a) standard prosthesis; (b) more tapered stem; (c) less tapered stem. P, prosthesis; CO, cortical bone; CA, cancellous bone; C, cement; PL, plateau (from Yettram and Wright, *J. Biomed. Engng.*, **1**, 282; reproduced by permission of Butterworth-Heinemann Ltd).

Crowninshield *et al.* (1980) have both presented three-dimensional models of the proximal implanted femur albeit still assuming linear elastic behaviour and isotropic properties for the materials. Indeed Rohlmann *et al.* (1983) remodelled their full femur (Rohlmann *et al.*, 1982) to include an implant which resulted in a system of 3663 hexahedral elements which generated more than 15 000 degrees of freedom (Figure 11.5). With this model they carried out a quite comprehensive parametric study of the structural behaviour, which they later extended to cover further aspects due to variations in stem design (Rohlmann *et al.*, 1987).

Also using a three-dimensional idealization, with over 6000 degrees of freedom, Fagan and Lee (1986) paid particular attention to the influence of a calcar collar on the stress distribution. With an even more detailed idealization involving 12 416 degrees of freedom, Prendergast *et al.* (1989) examined the effect of the stiffness of the stem material on the stem stresses and hence on the fatigue life of the prosthesis (Figure 11.6).

In practically all of the models referred to above the composite structure comprising bone, prosthesis and, where present, cement, were assumed to be fully monolithic, i.e. there was complete structural connection between the components at the interfaces. Thus all forms of stress – direct tensile, direct compressive and shear – could be transmitted across the junctions. In many situations *in vivo* this situation is not realistic in that in the case of a smooth-surfaced prosthesis and a conventional orthopaedic cement there is no bond. Normal tension cannot be transmitted across the interface and the shear carrying capability will depend upon the coefficient of friction.

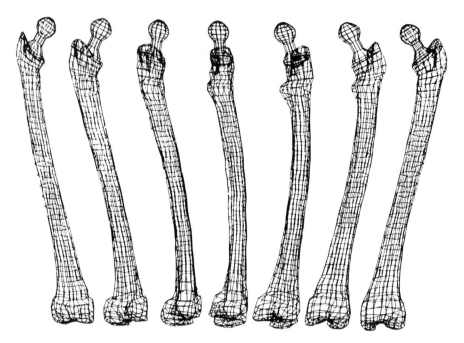

Figure 11.5 Various views of three-dimensional finite element mesh for whole femur with implanted prosthesis (from Rohlmann *et al.*, *J. Biomech.*, **16**, 731; reproduced by permission of Pergamon Press).

Likewise between the cement and the bone (or in the cementless case between the prosthesis and the bone) a layer of fibrous tissue builds up which has a major influence on the behaviour of the system. Where the surface is treated such as to encourage bony ingrowth to occur when cement is not used, or should an adhesive cement become available, then treating the interfaces as fully monolithic could be justified.

Improved treatment of the interfaces has attracted the attention of investigators in recent years although this aspect of the situation was noted much earlier. Svensson *et al.* (1976) noted that slip at the metal/cement junction could be simulated by removing elements of the cement where normal tensile stresses occurred, and carrying out an iterative analysis until convergence was obtained. Röhrle *et al.* (1977) also considered the possibility of tangential slippage between the prosthesis stem and the bone. Hampton and Andriacchi (1980) used a test for interface impingement at the junctions between elements of different components. In their three-dimensional model Brown *et al.* (1988) introduced a 'border zone' between the cement and the cancellous bone to which they assigned decreasing values of elastic modulus to represent its progressive decay. Rohlmann *et al.* (1988, 1989) have

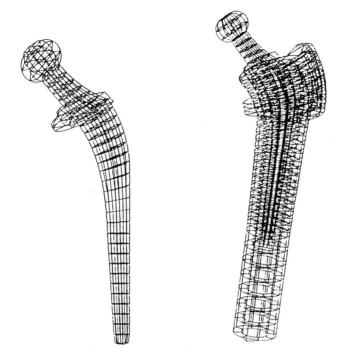

Figure 11.6 Three-dimensional finite element meshes for prosthesis and implanted proximal femur (from Prendergast *et al.*, *Clinical Materials*, **4**, 363; reproduced by permission of Elsevier Science Publishers Ltd).

investigated the non-monolithic contact situation using an iterative procedure and have tested it on a pseudo-implant, a circular cylindrical bar within cylindrical tubes and loaded as a cantilever.

There are various methods of representing a non-bonded interface with a finite-element model of a compound structure. Two of these are in common use for conventional engineering situations. These can be illustrated for the case of an interface across which compressive stress but not tensile stress can be transmitted. The first of these is by the incorporation of a non-linear spring element between corresponding nodes on each of the mating surfaces, these nodes being notionally coincident. This spring element has the property that its stiffness in tension is negligible whereas it is very high in compression. In the alternative approach the spring is omitted and the normal displacements at the corresponding nodes are compared. If these are such that the two components would appear to 'overlap' then the two nodes are coalesced to one; if they wish to move apart then a gap is allowed to open. Both these methods are clearly non-linear and an iterative procedure is required until the process settles down to a solution.

From a computing point of view, both approaches are therefore more expensive in resources than a simple fully monolithic analysis. The former is more economical in computer storage requirements but suffers from a practical difficulty in that the analyst must choose values of spring stiffness, both high and low, which do not adversely affect the mathematical conditioning of the system. The latter can be more expensive in computer storage but it avoids this problem. It was used by Yettram (1989) in conjunction with a two-dimensional model, incorporating a side plate, of a Freeman hip endoprosthesis. Prendergast and Taylor (1990) uncoupled the interface nodes locally between the collar and calcar in their three-dimensional simulation. The effect of the coefficient of friction between metal/cement and cement/bone in relation to the integrity of the interfaces has been studied by Clift and Miles (1990) using a finite element model of an axisymmetrical cone pushed into an initially matching conical hole. Using a two-dimensional model with a side plate, Weinans *et al.* (1990) investigated the behaviour of a total hip replacement with non-linear bonding characteristics, using an iterative procedure in reducing the stiffness of the interface layers to zero when no tension or shear occurred.

Reproducing accurately the geometry of a bone and its internal structure, both in its natural state and also when it includes an implant, in order to create a representative finite element model is not a particularly easy task. This has been achieved by various means, for example by using data from radiographs. For *in vitro* work a common procedure has been to implant a specimen into an acrylic block which is then sliced progressively along its length. The outline of bone within each slice is then digitized and a solid computer model reconstructed from these profiles. With the development of more sophisticated methods of medical imaging, such as computed tomography, and computer aided geometric modelling, more realistic finite element models can be produced. Both Marom and Linden (1990) and Keyak *et al.* (1990) have used CT scans for this purpose, the former actually for the tibia.

There is a multitude of different designs of hip replacement endoprostheses available on the market. Although there is general similarity between them they vary in detail in many respects such as ball diameter, stem shape, stem length, material and presence or absence of a collar. Added to this, some are for cemented application and others not, such as those of which the stems are hydroxyapatite coated. All the work which has been carried out into analysing the structural behaviour of the implanted prosthesis aims towards eventually producing a design which is the most satisfactory clinically as regards function (strength, stability and long life) and ease of insertion. Most of the investigations referred to above include parametric studies to determine how the various factors affect the overall performance. Again due

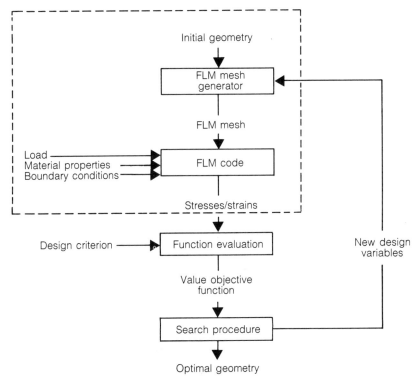

Figure 11.7 A global scheme for the FEM numerical shape optimization procedure (from Huiskes, R. and Boeklagen, R., *J. Biomech.*, **22**, 794; reproduced by permission of Pergamon Press).

to the availability of more powerful computers and the development of numerical methods, more sophisticated approaches are beginning to be employed for the design process. These are based upon sophisticated mathematical optimization techniques. At present they are just being employed on simplified systems, for example by Yoon *et al.* (1989) where the structural model is an axisymmetric nest of components and by Huiskes and Boeklagen (1989) where it is two-dimensional with side plate. In both these investigations the accent was on shape optimization of the prosthesis stem. No doubt as techniques and economic computer power develop they will be applied to other parameters, for example in the design of prostheses made from composite materials (Shirandami and Esat, 1990). It is interesting to compare this current approach to design illustrated by Huiskes and Boeklagen (1989), Figure 11.7, with that from Rybicki (1982), Figure 11.8.

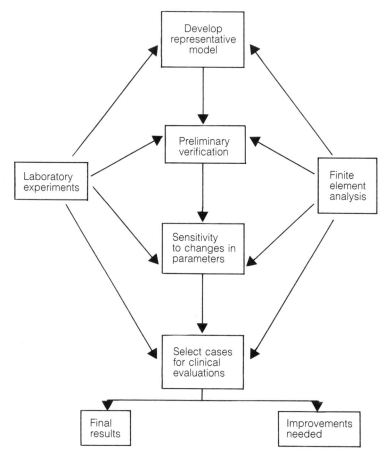

Figure 11.8 Interactions between finite element analysis, experiments and clinical evaluations (from Rybicki, E.F., in *Finite Elements in Biomechanics*, 1982, p. 186; reproduced by permission of John Wiley).

11.4 CONCLUSIONS

In this chapter a review of some of the major, but by no means all, attempts to analyse the stress and strain in the proximal femur, with or without an implanted endoprosthesis, has been presented. No attempt has been made to discuss the relative merits of each with respect to the results obtained. Some of the investigators have presented comparisons of their own results with *in vivo* experiments which they themselves have conducted. Each has used different forms of model with different idealizations involved. In some the femoral bone has been taken as isotropic and in others anisotropic and many diverse values have been used for the material properties. The loadings have varied to a large extent both in value and in form. Some analysts have merely used the hip-joint force to the head of the femur or prosthesis whilst others have included the forces in the abductor muscles to the greater trochanter and/or the ilio-psoas force. Two-dimensional, semi-three-dimensional and fully three-dimensional finite element models have been developed all based upon different femur geometries. Some have treated the system as fully monolithic whereas more recently the non-linear effect of the interfaces has been taken into account.

With this proliferation of different models and idealizations it is virtually impossible to assess the relative merits of each analysis or the validity of the approximations and assumptions which are inherent in them. What would appear to be needed is a comprehensive set of test results including measured forces, strains and displacements, with full geometric and material property data, from a series of fully instrumented experiments *in vitro*. These would need to cover a range of current prosthesis designs, both cemented and non-cemented. These data would serve as 'bench-marks' and would need to be available to all analysts so that the multitude of different procedures could be assessed one to another and to a common standard.

Total hip replacement based on the ball with endoprosthetic stem system as the femoral component is now a commonplace clinical procedure. The extensive effort which has been expended by many researchers, of whom those referenced herein are but a selected number, into its analysis as a load-bearing composite structure, has helped to make this form of treatment of diseased hips the great success which it undoubtedly has been. However, there is no analytical model in existence at this time which faithfully simulates all aspects of the real behaviour. But from extrapolation of the rate of progress from past developments, such a model may well become available in the not too distant future.

REFERENCES

Anand, S.C., Linder, J.L. and Moyle, D.D. (1978) Stress analysis of hip prostheses. *Proc. 31st ACEMB*, Atlanta, pp. 277.

Andriacchi, T.P., Galante, J.O., Belytschko, T.B. and Hampton, S. (1976) A stress analysis of the femoral stem in total hip prostheses. *J. Bone Jt. Surg.*, **58A**, 618–24.

Bartel, D.L. and Desormeaux, S.G. (1977) Femoral stem performance. *National Bureau of Standards Spec. Pub. 472*, pp. 51–9.

Brekelmans, W.A.M. and Poort, H.W. (1973) Theoretical and experimental investigation of the stress and strain situation on a femur. *Acta Orthop. Belg.*, **39** (1), 3–23.

Brown, T.D., Pedersen, D.R., Radin, E.L. and Rose, R.M. (1988) Global mechanical consequences of reduced cement/bone coupling rigidity in proximal femoral arthroplasty: a three dimensional finite element analysis. *J. Biomech.*, **21**, 115–29.

Brown, T.D., Way, M.E. and Ferguson, A.B. (1980) Stress transmission anomalies in femoral heads altered by aseptic necrosis. *J. Biomech.*, **13**, 687–99.

Carter, D.R., Orr, T.E. and Fyhrie, D.P. (1989) Relationships between loading history and femoral cancellous bone architecture. *J. Biomech.*, **22**, 231–44.

Clift, S.E. and Miles, A.W. (1990) A parametric finite-element analysis of the influence of the stem–cement interface in total hip replacement. *Proc. 7th Mtg Euro. Soc. Biomechs.*, Aarhus, A22.

Crowninshield, R.D., Brand, R.A., Johnston, R.C. and Milroy, J.C. (1980) An analysis of femoral component design in total hip arthroplasty. *J. Bone Jt. Surg.*, **62–A**, 68–78.

Fagan, M.J. and Lee, A.J.C. (1986) Role of the collar on the femoral stem of cemented total hip replacements. *J. Biomed. Engng.*, **8**, 295–304.

Fung, Y.C. (1981) Biomechanics, in *Mechanical Properties of Living Tissues*, Springer-Verlag, New York.

Fyhrie, D.P. and Carter, D.R. (1990) Femoral head apparent density distribution predicted from bone stresses. *J. Biomech.*, **23**, 1–10.

Gallagher, R.H., Simon, B.R., Johnson, P.C. and Gross, J.F. (1982) *Finite Elements in Biomechanics*, John Wiley, New York.

Gola, M.M. and Gugliotta, A.A. (1979) Analytical estimate of stresses in bones and prosthesis stems. *J. Strain Anal.*, **14**, 29–33.

Hampton, S.J. and Andriacchi, T.P. (1980) An analytical representation of the non-linear interface condition in a bone-cement-prosthesis system. *Proc. Int. Conf. on Finite Elements in Biomechanics* (ed. B.R. Simon), pp. 193–206.

Hampton, S.J., Andriacchi, T.P. and Galante, J.O. (1980) Three dimensional stress analysis of the femoral stem of a total hip prosthesis. *J. Biomech.*, **13**, 443–8

Hampton, S.J., Andriacchi, T.P., Galante, J.O. and Belytschko, T.B. (1976) Analytical approaches to the study of stresses in the femoral stem of total hip prostheses. *Proc. 29th ACEMB*, Boston, p. 244.

Huiskes, R. and Boeklagen, R. (1989) Mathematical shape optimization of hip prosthesis design. *J. Biomech.*, **22**, 793–804.

Keyak, J.H., Meagher, J.M., Skinner, H.B. and Mote, C.D. (1990) Automated three-dimensional finite element modelling of bone – A new method. *J. Biomed. Engng.*, **12**, 389–97.

Marom, S.A. and Linden, M.J. (1990) Computer aided stress analysis of long bones utilizing computed tomography. *J. Biomech.*, **23**, 399–404.

McNeice, G.M. (1975) Finite element studies of femoral endoprostheses for hip reconstruction. *Biomechanics Symposium*, ASME, AMD, Vol. 10, pp. 89–92.

NAFEMS (1986) *A Finite Element Primer*, Department of Trade and Industry, Glasgow.

Nath, B. (1974) *Fundamentals of Finite Elements for Engineers*, Athlone Press, London.

Piotrowski, G. and Wilcox, G.A. (1971) The stress program: a computer program for the analysis of stresses in long bones. *J. Biomech.*, **4**, 497–506.

Prendergast, P.J., Monaghan, J. and Taylor, D. (1989) Materials selection in the artificial hip joint using finite element stress analysis. *Clin. Mater.*, **4**, 361–76.

Prendergast, P.J. and Taylor, D. (1990) Stress analysis of the proximo-medial femur after total hip replacement. *J. Biomed. Engng.*, **12**, 379–82.

Raftopoulos, D.D. and Qassem, W. (1987) Three-dimensional curved beam stress analysis of the human femur. *J. Biomed. Engng.*, **9**, 356–66.

Rohlmann, A., Cheal, E.J., Hayes, W.C. and Bergmann, G. (1988) A non linear finite element analysis of interface conditions in porous coated hip endoprostheses. *J. Biomech.*, **21**, 605–11.

Rohlmann, A., Cheal, E.J., Hayes, W.C. and Bergmann, G. (1989) A non-linear finite element model for interface stresses in total hip replacements, in *Material Properties and Stress Analysis in Biomechanics* (Chapter 15) (ed. A.L. Yettram), Manchester University Press, Manchester.

Rohlmann, A., Mössner, U., Bergmann, G. and Kölbel, R. (1982) Finite-element-analysis and experimental investigation of stresses in a femur. *J. Biomed. Engng.*, **4**, 241–6.

Rohlmann, A., Mössner, U., Bergmann, G. and Kölbel, R. (1983) Finite-element-analysis and experimental investigation in a femur with hip endoprosthesis. *J. Biomech.*, **16**, 727–42.

Rohlmann, A., Mössner, U., Bergmann, G., Hees, G. and Kölbel, R. (1987) Effects of stem design and material properties on stresses in hip endoprostheses. *J. Biomed. Engng.*, **9**, 77–83.

Röhrle, H., Scholten, R., Sollbach, W., Ritter, G. and Grünert, A. (1977) Der Kraftfluss bei Hüftendoprothesen. *Arch. Orthop. Unfall-Chir.*, **89**, 49–60.

Rybicki, E.F. (1982) The role of finite element models in orthopaedics, in *Finite Elements in Biomechanics* Chapter 10, (eds R.H. Gallagher, B.R. Simon, P.C. Johnson and J.F. Gross), John Wiley, New York.

Rybicki, E.F., Simonen, F.A. and Weis, E.B. (1972) On the mathematical analysis of stress in the human femur. *J. Biomech.*, **5**, 203–15.

Shirandami, R. and Esat, I.I. (1990) New design of hip prosthesis using carbon fibre reinforced composite. *J. Biomed. Engng.*, **12**, 19–22.

Svensson, N.L., Valliappan, S. and Wood, R.D. (1976) Stress analysis of human femur with implanted Charnley prosthesis. Report No. 1976/AM/1, School of Mechanical and Industrial Engineering, University of New South Wales, Sydney.

Toridis, T.G. (1969) Stress analysis of the femur. *J. Biomech.*, **2**, 163–74.

Valliappan, S., Svensson, N.L. and Wood, R.D. (1977) Three dimensional stress analysis of the human femur. *Comput. Biol. Med.*, **7**, 253–64.

Weinans, H., Huiskes, R. and Grootenboer, H.J. (1990) Trends of mechanical consequences and modelling of a fibrous membrane around femoral hip prostheses. *J. Biomech.*, **23**, 991–1000.

Yamada, H. (1970) *Strength of Biological Materials*, Williams and Wilkins, Baltimore.

Yettram, A.L. (1989) Effect of interface conditions on the behaviour of a Freeman hip endoprothesis. *J. Biomed. Engng.*, **11**, 520–4.

Yettram, A.L. and Wright, K.W.J. (1979) Biomechanics of the femoral component of total hip prostheses with particular reference to the stress in the bone cement. *J. Biomed. Engng.*, **1**, 281–5.

Yettram, A.L. and Wright, K.W.J. (1980) Dependence of stem stress in total hip replacement on prosthesis and cement stiffness. *J. Biomed. Engng.*, **2**, 54–9.

Yoon, Y.S., Jang, G.H. and Kim, Y.Y. (1989) Shape optimal design of the stem of a cemented hip prosthesis to minimize stress concentration in the cement layer. *J. Biomech.*, **22**, 1279–84.

Zienkiewicz, O.C. (1989) *The Finite Element Method*, 4th edn, McGraw-Hill, London.

Index